Acoustics
for
Audiologists

A Singular Audiology Textbook
Jeffrey L. Danhauer, Ph.D.
Audiology Editor

Acoustics
for
Audiologists

Edgar Villchur, M.S.ed.

Foundation for Hearing Research
Woodstock, New York

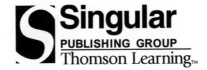

Singular Publishing Group
401 West A Street, Suite 325
San Diego, California 92101-7904

Singular Publishing Group, Inc., publishes textbooks, clinical manuals, clinical reference books, journals, videos, and multimedia materials on speech-language pathology, audiology, otorhinolaryngology, special education, early childhood, aging, occupational therapy, physical therapy, rehabilitation, counseling, mental health, and voice. For your convenience, our entire catalog can be accessed on our website at http://www.singpub.com. Our mission to provide you with materials to meet the daily challenges of the ever-changing health care/educational environment will remain on course if we are in touch with you. In that spirit, we welcome your feedback on our products. Please telephone (**1-800-521-8545**), fax (**1-800-774-8398**), or e-mail (singpub@singpub.com) your comments and requests to us.

© 2000, by Singular Publishing Group

Typeset in 10/12 Palatino by Black Dot Group
Printed in Canada by Webcom

All rights, including that of translation, reserved. No part of this publication may be reproduced, stored in a retrieval system or transmitted in any form or by any means, electronic, mechanical, recording, or otherwise, without the prior written permission of the publisher.

Library of Congress Cataloging-in-Publication Data

Villchur, Edgar.
   Acoustics for audiologists / by Edgar Villchur.
      p.   cm. — (A singular audiology textbook)
   Includes bibliographical references and index.
   ISBN 0-7693-0064-2 (soft cover : alk. paper)
   1. Audiology   2. Hearing disorders—Diagnosis.   3. Acoustics.
I. Title.   II. Series: Singular audiology text.
    [DNLM: 1. Acoustics.   2. Hearing—physiology.   3. Hearing
Disorders—physiopathology.   WV 270 V727a 2000]
RF291.V54   2000
617.8—DC21
DNLM/DLC
for Library of Congress   99-31869
                                                 CIP

Contents

Preface

A more accurate title for this book would be "Acoustics, Psychoacoustics, and Electronics for Audiologists," but that title is a little cumbersome, and most of the book is about acoustics.

In any case, this book is addressed to what I perceive as a need to include more physical science in current audiology training programs. It is written primarily for clinical audiologists or hearing-aid dispensers; audiology-research workers and hearing-aid designers need a more detailed, quantitative text. But sometimes an introductory text that discusses basic concepts qualitatively is useful even to the professionals in physical science, and may be consulted by them secretly.

Thirty-five years ago I wrote a similar basic book on the reproduction of sound. Some of the material of the present book inevitably overlaps that of the previous one, and something less than 10% of this book has been borrowed from my earlier work. Most of the illustrations are taken, with the generous permission of both authors and publishers, from published works. I have tried to use diagrams from the original disclosures relative to the subject: the ear-transmission curves of Shaw, Killion's illustration of horn design in hearing-aid tubing, and even a drawing of the Helmholtz resonator from Helmholtz' original 19th-century work.

Acknowledgment

It is both a duty and a pleasure to acknowledge the invaluable help of Professor Mead C. Killion, of Northwestern University and Etymotic Research, who with a friendly but rigorous eye scanned the manuscript, ruthlessly excised anything that seemed unclear or inaccurate, and suggested improvements.

Dedication
To Rosemary, Miriam, and Mark

CHAPTER I

The Sound Wave

The sound wave is an impulse, travelling in an elastic medium, that causes the particles of the medium to vibrate longitudinally, that is, back and forth along the path of travel. In the course of this vibration the particles alternately crowd together and spread apart, creating areas in which the medium is in turn compressed and rarified.

The source of sound is what Isaac Newton called a "tremulous body"—a vibrating string, diaphragm, or similar device—which first pushes the particles of air or other medium against one another, compressing the medium, and then draws back to form a slight rarefaction. Force applied to a rigid body would cause the whole body to move like a piston, all parts in unison, but an acoustic medium is elastic.[1] Particles in the area of intensified pressure exert a repelling force on particles further from the source, making them in turn crowd together, and the pressure area moves out with a predetermined velocity from the original disturbance; the rarified air exerts a pulling force on neighboring molecules further from the source, and in bringing these in to fill the partial vacuum creates a new rarefaction farther out. Thus a wave moves out from the source, but the particles of the transmission

[1]An acoustic medium is elastic when stimulated at audio frequencies, but may act as a rigid body when stimulated at lower frequencies. For example, a free steel bar will conduct a longitudinal sound wave, but move like a rigid piston when a steady longitudinal force (without torsional or transverse components) is applied at one end.

medium only vibrate and never get anywhere. It is the disturbance of the medium, not the medium itself, that travels away from the source. The speed of sound in air at 68°F (20°C) is approximately 1127 ft/ second (344 m/s).

If we were to analyze the pressure state of the medium a short while after the source of sound had started to vibrate, we would see a condition such as that illustrated in Figure 1–1A. This diagram represents the pressure state pictorially. The condition of the medium may also be represented symbolically by a graph, as in Figure 1–1B, in which points of maximum pressure are recorded by the graph peaks, points of normal atmospheric pressure by crossings of the horizontal axis, and points of maximum rarefaction by the graph troughs.

In the 17th century Robert Boyle demonstrated that the transmission of sound cannot take place without a physical medium. He suspended a bell in an evacuated glass jar, and when the bell was rung the sound was inaudible. Before the moon was visited, one feature of its airless environment was already known: There would be no sound except for vibrations transmitted through the solid surface.

When a stone is dropped into a pool of water, waves travel out in all directions, a phenomenon often used as an analogy to the action of

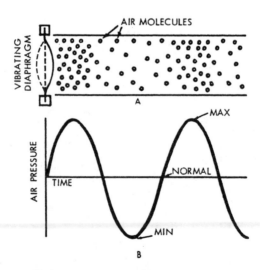

Figure 1–1. A. Alternate compression and rarefaction of air created by a sound wave. **B.** The pressure condition of the air molecules in A represented symbolically by a graph. (From *Reproduction of Sound*, by E. Villchur, 1965, p. 2. New York: Dover Publications. Reprinted with permission.)

sound waves. The force of the dropped stone is sent out through the water, but as in the case of sound, the particles merely vibrate in orderly sequence and do not travel with the force. There is an important difference, however, between this type of wave motion and that of sound. The particles of water vibrate up and down, in a direction approximately transverse to the direction of wave travel, rather than back and forth along the path of the wave. The mechanical water wave is thus called *transverse*, a sound wave *longitudinal*.

A transverse wave may be represented in a graph by a cross-sectional view of the medium along the path of the wave. A pattern of the wave is created in space by the instantaneous position of the vibrating particles, because the particles vibrate across rather than with the direction of wave travel. But sound waves do not look like their representations in graph form.

The symbolic representation of a sound wave by a graph facilitates an analysis of the qualities of the sound. A listener would never mistake a bass drum for an oboe, but the differences can also be displayed on an oscilloscope and stated in quantitative terms. There are four basic physical characteristics of sound, as illustrated in Figure 1–2: the amplitude of the pressure swings, the frequency of the vibration, the shape of the waveform, and the shape of the wave envelope. These physical characteristics are primarily associated, in that order, with the sensations of loudness, pitch, timbre, and the sensation—for which there is no single word—created by short-term amplitude changes, such as amplitude vibrato and the transient effects at the starting and stopping of a sound.

AMPLITUDE AND LOUDNESS

The greater the vertical distance between the peak and the trough of the graph of a sound wave, the more the air is being compressed and rarefied, the greater the vibration impressed on the eardrum, and the greater the intensity of the sound. This characteristic is called *amplitude*. The amplitude of sound is expressed in units of pressure, intensity, or power.

Pressure is the force per unit area exerted on the medium perpendicular to the path of the wave, measured in microbars (μbar) or the older, equivalent dynes per square centimeter (dyne/cm^2). A microbar is one millionth of a bar; a bar is approximately the pressure of 1 (0.98697) standard atmosphere.

Intensity is the energy transmitted by the sound wave per unit of area, measured in watts/cm^2. The term intensity takes into consideration both pressure and the energy transmitted by the medium; for a

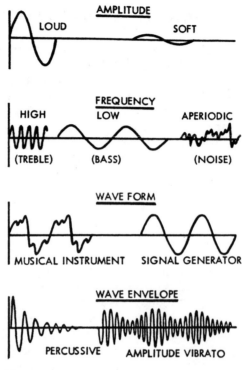

Figure 1-2. Four physical characteristics of sound. (From *Reproduction of Sound*, by E. Villchur, 1965, p. 4. New York: Dover Publications. Reprinted with permission.)

given medium, either pressure or intensity may be used to represent amplitude. The term intensity is also used in a general sense, as an expression to distinguish the physical amplitude of sound from its loudness.

Neither of these terms count the total area over which the sound is spread. When we count the area (perpendicular to the direction of travel) serviced, or are concerned with the total output of the source, we use a third term, *power*. Power is the energy transmitted per second, measured in *watts*.

The term that describes our perception of sound amplitude is *loudness*. It corresponds primarily to the physical characteristic of amplitude, but loudness is also influenced by other characteristics such as frequency and duration, and will be discussed in more detail in Chapter 6.

FREQUENCY AND PITCH

Frequency is the number of times per second a complete sequence of the vibratory event called a *cycle* occurs: from rest, to maximum pressure or displacement, through rest again, to minimum pressure or displacement, and back to rest. The number of cycles per second, formerly called cycles/ or cps, is now referred to as *Hertz (Hz)*. The sensation of pitch depends on it, although pitch is also influenced by other factors such as amplitude. The greater the number of Hz, the higher the pitch.

The reciprocal of the frequency is the number of seconds per cycle; 1 second divided by the frequency in Hz is the time taken up by 1 cycle and is called a *period*.

The *wavelength* of a sound, conventionally represented by the Greek letter lambda (λ), is the distance along the path of travel covered by one cycle: for example, from a point in space at which maximum compression takes place to the corresponding point of the cycle ahead. Figure 1–3, from Moore (1997), plots the sound-pressure variations of a wave against time, with the period labeled. If the pressure variations had been plotted against distance along the path of the wave rather than against time, the distance along the horizontal axis of the graph labeled "period" would then represent the wavelength.

The distance sound travels in 1 second divided by the number of cycles in that second is the distance traveled during 1 cycle, or the

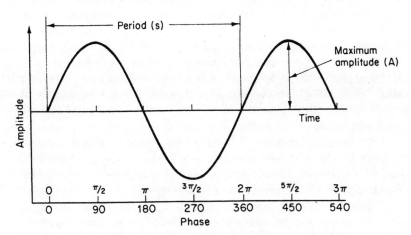

Figure 1–3. The phase and period of a sine wave. If the progress of the vibration were plotted against distance of travel rather than time, the section labeled "period" would be the wavelength. (From *An Introduction to the Psychology of Hearing,* by B. C. J. Moore, 1997, p. 2. New York: Academic Press. Reprinted with permission.)

wavelength. Because the distance traveled in 1 second defines speed and the number of cycles in one second defines frequency, the speed of sound divided by the frequency is the wavelength.

In formal terms the wavelength, the frequency, the period, and the speed of sound are related as follows:

$$\lambda = V/f = V \times p$$

where λ = wavelength in feet

V = speed of sound = 1127 ft/s in air at 68°F

f = frequency in Hz

p = period in seconds

For example, the wavelength of a 1–kHz tone is equal to the speed of sound in ft/s divided by the frequency in Hz: 1127/1000, or 1.127 ft (0.344 m); the wavelength of a 100 Hz tone is 1127/100, or 11.27 ft.

Nonperiodic Sound

All sounds do not have pitch: The presence of a definite pitch requires that a number of successive cycles of the same frequency be repeated. Regularity of this nature makes the sound a *periodic* one.

Nonperiodic sound is produced by sources of sound such as automobiles or leaves in the wind and is referred to as noise. Noise is also created by an electronic noise generator, whose output contains a mix of all the audio frequencies. This mix may be shaped to conform to the frequency distribution of energy in typical speech, in which case it is called speech-shaped noise and contains a broad suggestion of pitch. If the generator noise is designed to have equal energy per octave, it is called *"pink noise"*; if it has equal energy per cycle, it is called *"white noise."* White noise is and sounds like noise with high-frequency emphasis, because each higher frequency octave in the frequency spectrum has twice the number of cycles as the previous octave. Pink noise is closer to, but not the same as, speech-shaped noise. *Narrow-band noise*—for example, noise whose frequency spectrum is one third of an octave wide—is sometimes used as a test signal.

White noise has on occasion been used in testing hearing-impaired subjects for speech intelligibility in noise, but its concentration of energy at high frequencies makes it inappropriate for that use, for two reasons. First, the frequency distribution of energy in white noise is not representative of the interference encountered in real life; and second, typical hearing-impaired subjects have their greatest loss at high frequencies. Subjects are likely to hear white noise at greatly reduced levels relative to speech. Villchur (1977) showed that white noise was much less effective than speech-spectrum noise in reducing speech intelligibility in cases of high-frequency loss.

The current musical standard for middle A is 440 Hz. The frequency range of audible sound for a young person with normal hearing is about 20 Hz to 20,000 Hz (20 kHz), although this range is strongly dependent on the level of the test sounds.

WAVEFORM AND TIMBRE

The graph of an individual cycle of a sound wave, called its *waveform*, includes information about all of the frequency components of the sound, which in combination primarily determine its timbre or tone color. The waveform in Figure 1–1 is that of a sound created by the simplest of vibrations. It has only one frequency component, and it is called a sine wave because it is a plot of the mathematical sine function.[2] It is found relatively rarely in nature, and has little interest musically. The tone produced by blowing across the top of a bottle, except for the noise component, is of this type; and sine waves are, of course, produced by an electronic sine-wave generator. Sine waves are the most common type of signal used in audiometric measurements, because they make it possible to test a subject's response to a single-frequency signal that provides no stimuli at other frequencies.

The timbre of a musical instrument is associated with a waveform shape that is almost never sinusoidal and that is characteristic of its musical sound. Musical instruments and the human voice mechanism —singing or speaking—vibrate in complex ways, both as a whole and in sections. In addition to producing sound at the frequency corresponding to the note in the musical score, they simultaneously produce sound at many other, higher frequencies. The basic tone that identifies the pitch of the sound is called the *fundamental,* while the higher frequency components are called *overtones;* the term *partial* refers to any component of a sound, fundamental or overtone. It is the particular combination of fundamental and overtones, in number, kind, and relative amplitude that determines the waveform and the timbre of a sound.

Figure 1–4, from Seashore's early study on the perception of music (1938), shows the waveform of the musical tone of a violin, made up of

---

[2]If the sine of an angle is plotted against values of the angle from 0° to 360°, the resulting graph is one cycle of a sine wave.

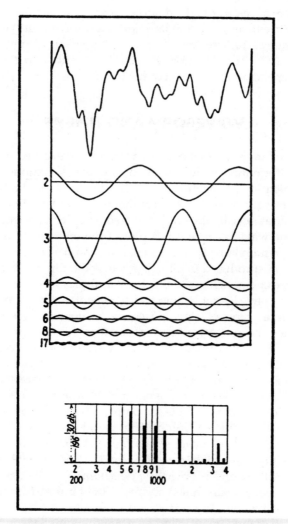

Figure 1-4. Above: waveform and harmonic composition of a violin tone (G below middle C). The fundamental, the lowest-frequency component, is 196 Hz. Below: the same information presented in a line spectrum. (From *Psychology of Music,* by C. E. Seashore, 1938, p. 98. New York: McGraw-Hill Book Company.)

a combination of its fundamental and its overtones. No matter how many frequency components there are in a sound, each molecule of the medium can have only one position at a given moment, and the pressure state of the medium at that moment and at a given point in space can have only one value. The single curve of the violin waveform thus represents the complex sound of the violin, and we hear its many components simultaneously as a single sound. The same information about the violin sound is given in the lower diagram of Figure 1–4, which is in the form of a *line spectrum*. The height of each bar represents the amplitude of the component of sound at that frequency.

In most musical instruments the overtone frequencies are whole multiples of the fundamental frequency. Such overtones are called *harmonics*. The fundamental tone in Figure 1–4 is G below middle C, 196 Hz; therefore the second harmonic is 392 Hz, the third harmonic 588 Hz, and so forth.

The relative loudness of each frequency component of a complex tone is affected by the overall amplitude of the tone (see the equal-loudness contours in Chapter 6, Figure 6–1), so that the timbre of a sound, while determined primarily by its waveform, is affected by changes in overall amplitude. Turning down the volume of a radio reduces the apparent contribution of low-frequency components.

The harmonics, in addition to determining the timbre of the sound, reinforce the listener's sense of pitch. The difference between adjacent harmonics is always the fundamental frequency, and one way we identify pitch is to recognize the harmonic structure and respond to the difference frequency between harmonics: note that the fundamental violin tone in Figure 1–3 is not even a significant part of the sound. The recognition of pitch from the harmonic structure explains how, when we listen to a pocket radio that is incapable of reproducing low-frequency tones, we can still identify the pitch of the bass notes of a pipe organ or cello coming from that radio. One of my experimental hearing-impaired subjects, whose pitch discrimination had been affected, reported improved pitch discrimination when she was given hearing aids that restored the higher frequency harmonics of music to her hearing.

Not all musical instruments have overtones that are harmonic. Some instruments simultaneously produce such a varied assortment of harmonically unrelated overtones that they do not create a definite sensation of pitch. Strike tones and nonharmonic overtones make up a large part of the sound of such members of the percussive group as the triangle, the bass drum, and cymbals. In speech, the fricative sounds are grouped in the high-frequency region but do not have a regular harmonic pattern and do not have pitch (unless the speaker has a whistling /s/).

PHASE

The instantaneous *phase* of a sound refers to the condition of compression or rarefaction at a particular moment or at a particular point along the path of travel. Instantaneous phase is represented on the graph of an individual cycle of the sound wave by the position along the time or distance axis. The graph of Figure 1–3 shows the phase of a sound wave at different points along the horizontal axis, in degrees and in radians (π radians = 180°).

We may also refer to the overall phase of a periodic sound. Overall phase is represented in a graph by the left-right position of the wave along a horizontal time or distance axis. Overall phase is used in describing a general phase shift or in comparing the phase of one sound with that of another. Two sound waves of the same frequency are said to be in phase if their peaks and troughs occur at the same points on the horizontal axis, which is to say at the same points in time or space, and to be 180° out of phase if the peaks of one coincide with the troughs of the other. Sounds that are in phase reinforce each other; sounds that are out of phase cancel each other. The waveform of the violin tone of Figure 1–4 is formed by the combination of fundamental and harmonics shown at the lower part of the diagram, but if the phase of these components relative to one another were changed, the shape of the total waveform would also change.

Helmholtz (1885) concluded from his experiments that the subjective quality of a compound tone depends solely on the number and relative amplitude of its components and is independent of the relative phase of its components. Some later experimenters have reported that relative phase does have an effect on tone quality, but it is not likely that such an effect is of practical importance. The sounds of a symphony orchestra or of a string quartet are combined in what is essentially random phase determined by the musicians' seating arrangement and the position of the listening seat in the hall. The phase of any sound from any of the instruments is reversed, from peak to trough, every half wavelength of travel from the source. The wavelength of a 55-Hz fundamental tone (*A*) from a cello is 1127/55, or 20.5 ft., so that the phase of this fundamental is reversed every 10.25 feet of travel across the audience. The phase of a harmonic of *A* at 2750 Hz from a nearby violin is reversed every 2.5 inches of travel. The relative phase between the two sounds is a matter of chance: the phase of the higher frequency tone is subject to a turn of the listener's head or small movements by the player holding the instrument, either of which could change the phase relationship between the low- and high-frequency tones by 180°.

The characteristic of phase relates to hearing aids when sounds of the same frequency reinforce or cancel each other because of their relative phase, as in standing-wave air-column resonances (see Chapter 3), or in directional microphones (see Chapter 10). The difference in phase between the sound entering left and right ears is part of the binaural effect in hearing.

WAVE ENVELOPE

The wave envelope represents overall amplitude changes such as the swelling and fading of sound, amplitude vibrato, or a percussive attack followed by a slow decay. In speech, the instantaneous changes of amplitude within words, or the brief silence between /s/ and /t/ in a word like *stay*, are displayed in the wave envelope.

Some earlier record players were able to play records backwards, and could be used to demonstrate the importance of the wave envelope to sound quality. With attack and decay of the sound of a piano reversed, the piano sounds like a small organ or accordion with peculiar tone endings. Speech not only loses its intelligibility but changes its national character. English may sound like some unidentified foreign language because of the reversal of wave-envelope and pitch-intonation sequences.

The sound quality of a musical instrument, which we describe in subjective terms such as "fiery," "melancholy," or "brilliant," can also be described in terms of the four physical characteristics of sound referred to above. These characteristics describe speech as well, but the characteristics of speech that determine recognition require further analysis, and will be discussed separately in Chapter 7.

References

Helmholtz, H. (1954). 1885 English translation; 1954 reprint. *On the sensations of tone* (pp. 119–126). New York: Dover Publications.

Moore, B. C. J. (1997). *An introduction to the psychology of hearing* (p. 2). London: Academic Press.

Seashore, C. E. (1938). *Psychology of music* (p. 96). New York: McGraw-Hill Book Co.

Villchur, E. (1965). *Reproduction of sound* (pp. 2–4). New York: Dover Publications.

Villchur, E. (1977). Electronic models to simulate the effect of sensory distortions on speech perception by the deaf. *Journal of the Acoustical Society of America, 62*, 665–674.

CHAPTER 2

The Measurement of Sound: Octaves and Bels

THE FREQUENCY SCALE

Musical frequency intervals—the octave, halftone, etc.—and units of sound-power or electrical-power differences—the bel and decibel—have the same mathematical design. The first represents ratios of frequency, the second ratios of power.

A piano keyboard seems to be divided up evenly as far as pitch is concerned. The same apparent rise in pitch is produced by going from middle C to the next higher C and then to the C following, or from C to C-sharp to D. The first of these musical intervals is called an *octave*, the second a *half tone*. From C to D is a *whole tone*.

These apparently even increments of pitch do not correspond to similarly uniform physical increments in frequency. To increase the pitch by an octave, we do not add a given number of Hz but rather multiply the frequency by two. Starting at 440 Hz (A), one octave up takes us to 880 Hz; two octaves up takes us not to 1320 Hz (880 + 440) but to 1760 Hz (880 × 2). Any musical interval represents a *ratio* between frequencies rather than a given number of Hz. An octave at the bottom of a piano keyboard covers only 27.5 Hz, while an octave at the top of the keyboard covers 2093 Hz, but the range of musical pitch is the same for each octave because that is the way we perceive sound.

The frequency scale of a graph that is used to plot frequency-response curves or audiograms is designed to reflect this perception mode for pitch differences; the scale is graduated in frequency ratios rather than frequency increments. Figure 2–1 illustrates the similarity in layout between a piano keyboard and the frequency scale of the "logarithmic" form of graph used in audio engineering and in audiology. Figure 2–2 shows the contrast between a logarithmic graph and one with a linear (arithmetic) horizontal scale.

THE POWER SCALE

The way we hear changes in loudness is similar to the way we hear changes in pitch: perceived quantitative changes are more accurately represented by the ratio of the physical quantities than by their arithmetic differences. We therefore use a scale of amplitude—the decibel (dB) scale—that is in keeping with this mode of perception. The value of each unit in that scale is increased to that of the next higher unit by multiplying the value of the lower unit by a constant factor, creating a geo-

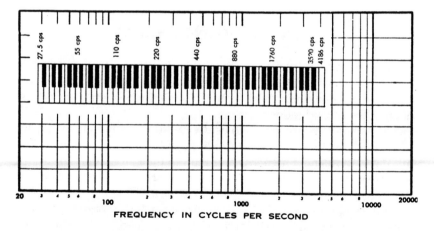

Figure 2–1. Comparison between a piano keyboard and a graph used to plot audio frequency-response curves. Both the keyboard and the horizontal scale of the graph (or of an audiogram) are laid out in frequency ratios. (From *Reproduction of Sound*, by E. Villchur, 1965, p. 6. New York: Dover Publications. Reprinted with permission.)

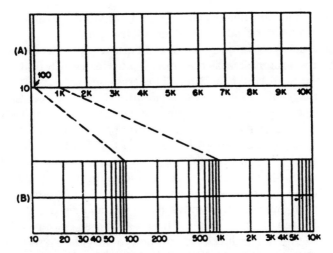

Figure 2-2. Comparison between linear (arithmetic) and logarithmic (geometric) frequency scales. **A.** Linear scale from 10 to 10,000 Hz. **B.** Logarithmic scale for the same frequency range. (From *Handbook of Sound Reproduction*, by E. Villchur, 1957, p. 8. Mineola, New York: Radio Magazines. Reprinted with permission.)

metric progression (e.g., 10, 100, 1000), rather than by adding a fixed amount, which would create an arithmetic progression (e.g., 10, 20, 30).

We could construct in our mind's eye a special keyboard instrument in which all keys played the same frequency, and ascending the "scale" increased only the intensity of the sound. This hypothetical instrument could be calibrated in decibels by designing it so that each adjacent higher key multiplied the sound power by an equal factor, a factor that made every 10 keys increase the power 10 times. For example, if .01 watt were produced by a given key, 10 keys further up would produce .1 watt, and 10 keys further, 1 watt. Each group of 10 keys would then correspond to a power ratio of 1 bel, and each adjacent key would increase the power by 1 decibel.

The horizontal frequency scale of the graph in Figure 2–1, as we have seen, follows a geometric progression. Because the units used for the horizontal frequency scale are not geometric octaves or semitones but Hz, which are linear, the horizontal scale must be laid out in geometric progression. The vertical scale of amplitude used in audiology also represents a geometric progression, but unlike the horizontal frequency scale it uses units of geometric ratio: decibels, not microbars. It is therefore laid out in arithmetic progression; the geometric progression of the amplitude scale is intrinsic in its dB units. If the amplitude scale were in linear units of sound pressure it would, like the frequency scale, have to be laid out in geometric progression. A scale in absolute units of sound pressure or of frequency (μbar or Hz), laid out in geometric progression, is the equivalent of a scale in units of decibels or octaves laid out in arithmetic progression.

The range of audible sound amplitudes, and the corresponding range of electrical voltages and power levels, is very great. In the frequency region of greatest hearing sensitivity, human ears can detect changes of sound pressure of the order of 0.0002 μbar, which is one five-billionth of normal atmospheric pressure; the average sound pressure of conversational speech is about two thousand times the sound pressure at the midrange-frequency hearing thresholds of normal listeners, and symphonic crescendos reach sound pressure levels more than a hundred thousand times the pressures at hearing threshold. The decibel unit of amplitude, in addition to providing a scale more or less in keeping with the way we hear changes in loudness, makes it possible to work with a much more convenient range of numbers.

Here are some simple definitions: a *bel* is a power ratio—normally of acoustical or electrical power—of 10 to 1; a *decibel* is a power ratio of 1.2589 to 1.

Decibel Math

Why that particular odd number of 1.2589?

Returning briefly to musical intervals will help put the question into perspective. In Western music, 12 successive half tones make an octave, a frequency ratio of 2 to 1. The frequency in Hz of each succeeding half tone in the tempered scale[1] has the same ratio to the tone preceding it, 1.0594631 to 1, an increase of just under 6%; when you multiply the frequency of each of 12 successive half tones by that number you get a ratio of 2 to 1 between the frequencies of the first and last tones, or a frequency range of one octave. In more formal mathematical terms, multiplying the frequency of a tone 12 times successively by the twelfth root of 2 ($\sqrt[12]{2} = 1.0594631$) doubles the frequency.

---

[1] In the tempered scale, the frequency ratio between any two adjacent halftones is the same, and the harmonics of different notes that would coincide in a "natural" or "just" scale miss by a small amount. Equal temperament, however, makes it possible for a keyboard instrument to play in any musical key without retuning. Bach's "Well-Tempered Clavier," a set of preludes and fugues for keyboard instrument in successive musical keys, marked his acceptance of the tempered scale.

As we have seen, the dB scale of power, like the musical scale, is a progression based on a multiplying factor rather than the addition of a fixed quantity. Ten successive 1-decibel increases make 1 bel, which is a power ratio of 10 to 1. When you multiply 10 successive values of power by 1.2589 you get a ratio of 10 to 1 between the first and last values, or a dynamic range of 1 bel; the power in watts of each succeeding 1-dB step is 1.2589 times the power of the preceding step. Multiplying a number 10 times successively by the tenth root of 10 ($\sqrt[10]{10} = 1.2589$) is the same as multiplying the number by 10.

Power Versus Sound Pressure or Voltage

The audiologist normally deals with units of sound pressure or voltage rather than of power. Acoustical or electrical power varies as the square of the sound pressure or voltage: if you double the voltage across a given load you quadruple the power, which is a power increase of 6 dB.[2] Since increasing the voltage is counted in terms of the effect on the power, the voltage only has to be doubled, not quadrupled, for a 6-dB increase. If we say sound power has been increased 6 dB, or the sound pressure has been increased 6 dB, it is the same thing; In either case the sound pressure has been doubled and the sound power has been quadrupled.

On the other hand, if sound pressure and sound power in absolute units are each multiplied by the same factor, the dB increase of pressure is not the same as the dB increase of power. Doubling the sound pressure is an increase of 6 dB, while doubling the sound power (which would mean the pressure had been increased by the square root of two) is an increase of only 3 dB. A tenfold increase of pressure or voltage is an increase of 20 dB or 2 bels, while a tenfold increase of power is an increase of 10 dB or 1 bel. A decibel may be counted as either a power ratio of 1.2589 to 1, or its equivalent, a voltage or sound-pressure ratio of 1.12202 ($\sqrt[20]{10}$) to 1: A 1 dB increase of sound amplitude is thus about a 12% increase of sound pressure and a 26% increase of power.

To convert the ratio between two values of power W_1 and W_2 to decibels:

$$\text{no. of dB} = 10 \log \frac{W_1}{W_2}$$

[2]To quadruple any value is the same as multiplying it by 1.2589 six times successively; quadrupling the power is thus a 6-dB increase.

To convert the ratio between two values of voltage, current, or pressure E_1 and E_2, in or across a given load, to decibels:

$$\text{no. of dB} = 20 \log \frac{E_1}{E_2}$$

The use of logarithms makes it practical and convenient to convert linear ratios to decibel units, but logarithms are only a calculating tool and not intrinsic to the definition of a decibel. A power ratio in linear units may be expressed in decibel units without using logarithms, with the equally accurate but much less convenient expression:

$$\frac{W_1}{W_2} = 1.2589^x,$$

where $x = $ the number of dB representing the ratio of $\dfrac{W_1}{W_2}$

Without logarithms, this equation cannot be solved for the value of x except by trial and error. However, an x number of decibels can be converted to a linear power ratio by raising 1.2589 to the power of x.

Decibel Values That Define Levels

The decibel has no absolute value, and is meaningless unless it refers to two values. It is like the expression "double" or "triple"; an unknown quantity cannot be defined as double unless we know what it is the double of. Yet sometimes decibel values seem to be used in absolute terms. For example, the level of typical conversational speech is described as being about 65 dB *sound-pressure level (SPL)*. Use of the term "level" indicates that the unit of measurement relates to some known reference, one which may be so well understood that it does not need to be stated explicitly. An SPL of 65 dB refers to sound pressure 65 dB above the standard reference sound pressure of 0.0002 microbar.

HEARING LEVEL

Audiometer ouput dials used to be calibrated in units of *hearing loss*; the numbers on the dial represented the difference between the output SPL of the audiometer and the threshold SPL of an average unimpaired listener, at the same frequency and with the same earphone. ANSI Standard S3.20-1973 now says the term hearing loss is "deprecated," and has substituted a term with the same meaning at threshold, *hearing level (HL)*.

The ANSI Standard defines hearing level as the SPL of the audiometer signal relative to the audiometer reference SPL at a specified frequency. A more general definition of threshold hearing level would be the number of dB a patient's threshold SPL exceeds normal threshold SPL at a particular frequency, assuming the conditions of measurement are the same for both patient thresholds and normal thresholds. SPLs other than threshold SPLs may be expressed in HLs—for example, to define presentation levels—by the same formula, that is, by subtracting normal threshold SPLs from the suprathreshold SPLs. Like sound-pressure levels, hearing levels are stated as a single decibel value that is really the ratio in dB to an implied reference, in this case normal threshold SPLs, which vary with frequency. The HL unit is simply the number of dB above normal threshold.

Normal hearing thresholds in HLs are the reference to which abnormal thresholds are related, and are by definition 0-dB HL at any frequency. The amount of hearing loss of a hearing-impaired person at each frequency is represented in an audiogram as the number of dB below this 0-dB reference (the vertical HL scale of an audiogram puts 0 dB at the top), and is defined as the *hearing threshold level (HTL)*. The reader is allowed to think of HTL as hearing threshold *loss*.

Normal thresholds expressed in SPLs, on the other hand, are the minimum physical sound pressures, in dB re 0.0002 μbar, at which an average unimpaired person hears sound at particular frequencies and under particular conditions. The values of these threshold SPLs depend on whether they are equivalent-coupler or real-ear SPLs, whether they are for binaural or monaural listening, and whether they represent *minimum audible pressure (MAP) or minimum audible field (MAF)*.

MAP refers to minimum audible sound pressure at the eardrum of the listener taking the threshold test. Sivian and White (1933), who proposed the term, meant eardrum sound pressure whatever the source of sound, but ANSI Standard S3.20-1973 specifies that the signals for MAP measurements must be presented by an earphone. The significance of the ANSI limitation is that most audiometer earphones create an increase of physiological-noise masking and raise thresholds in the frequency region below 500 Hz by up to 6 dB.

Like MAP, MAF refers to minimum audible sound pressure at the listener's position, but in an MAF measurement the listener must face the source of sound in a free field during the threshold test, and the point of measurement of the sound pressure is not the eardrum but the center of the listener's head, fortunately after the listener is removed. MAF threshold SPLs are lower than MAP threshold SPLs because external sound signals, unlike signals at the eardrum, have gain ahead of them before they get to the eardrum: They have yet to be subjected to the acoustic gain of the head and ear. This acoustic gain is illustrated in Shaw's (1974) data of Figure 5–1 in Chapter 5.

It was once thought that free-field hearing-threshold SPLs measured at the eardrum were lower by about 6 dB than earphone hearing thresholds measured at the same eardrum. Killion (1978), in a survey and analysis of previous studies, showed that the "missing 6 dB" existed only at low frequencies, where it was caused by physiological noise induced by the earphone. Outside of this effect, the free-field and earphone hearing thresholds measured at the eardrum proved to be the same, an unremarkable result. Killion commented: "It is no surprise that threshold occurs at a constant eardrum pressure."

Equivalent Threshold Sound-Pressure Level

Facilities for free-field measurements, or probe-tube microphones to measure eardrum sound pressures, are not among the ordinary tools of the audiologist. In clinical audiology, therefore, the values of normal threshold SPLs that provide the reference at each audiometer frequency for hearing levels (loss) have been established indirectly. The first step in that procedure was to determine the voltage across a specified earphone that produced threshold SPL at particular frequencies for an average normal listener. The values of these voltages alone are sufficient to establish normal threshold references with that earphone, and the actual threshold SPLs do not have to be known. However, in order to make it possible to transfer these data to other earphone models, and to check the acoustical calibration of the system, the earphone was placed on a specified coupler (artificial ear), and the previously measured threshold voltages at each frequency—plus some fixed amount which was later subtracted—was applied to the earphone. The SPLs created in the coupler by the earphone, called *equivalent threshold sound pressure levels*, serve as the normal-threshold reference SPLs. Different couplers and audiometer earphones are used in different countries, so different values of equivalent threshold SPLs have had to be established. They are listed in ISO Recommendation R/389-1964. Because audiometers are calibrated relative to equivalent threshold SPLs, the calibration of an audiometer is valid only for a particular earphone unless a correction is applied.

A subject's threshold SPLs minus normal threshold SPLs, a difference in dB that defines the subject's impairment in HLs, remains constant whether the threshold measurements are MAF, MAP, or equivalent coupler SPLs[3], but only if conditions for the subject measurements are the same as for the reference measurements. We cannot, for example, use equivalent coupler threshold SPLs as the normal reference for a subject's MAP threshold SPLs measured with a probe microphone. The hearing levels recorded in an audiogram are based on equivalent coupler measurements for both patient and reference threshold SPLs, and (except for earphone-induced noise) should match MAF- or MAP-derived hearing levels. MAF rather than equivalent coupler measurements are useful for comparing aided to unaided thresholds.

To convert audiogram values from HLs to SPLs—for the purpose of comparing the audiogram values to a speech band plotted in SPLs, for example, as in Figure 7–4 of Chapter 7 or Figure 9–1 of Chapter 9—normal-threshold SPLs are added to the HLs, and the vertical scale of the audiogram is reversed so that zero dB is at the bottom rather than at the top of the scale. While HLs are the same for different types of measurement, threshold SPLs are not, and the conversion factor from HL to SPL depends on whether we are looking for MAF, MAP, or equivalent coupler SPLs. Table 2–1 lists the conversion values to change audiogram HLs to MAF SPLs, the latter suitable for comparison to free-field speech SPLs. These values are derived from the ISO (1961) MAF normal binaural thresholds in SPLs, modified for monaural listening by adding 3 dB to the ISO thresholds.

The level of a sine-wave signal may be stated in either SPLs or HLs without ambiguity. It is another matter to measure the level of speech, which is made up of a variety of sound components at different frequencies, many of which occur simultaneously, and whose combined level varies from moment to moment. Speech audiometers that conform to ASA Standard C16.5 (1961) use a *volume unit (vu)* meter to monitor speech levels. The vu meter has standard mechanical and electrical characteristics, and speech levels are read as the maximum deflections over 1 minute, excluding one or two deflections of unusual magnitude.

When the many simultaneous components of speech are combined, the average speech level in SPL is about 15 dB higher than in HL. One reason for this large difference is that most of the time speech energy is concentrated at the lower frequencies (see Figure 7–4).

Although hearing thresholds can be specified in different units, the differences only have to do with the way the thresholds are measured and calibrated. All of the units represent the same phenomenon and the same hearing loss.

---

[3]I find that sometimes confusion about threshold HLs is cleared up by thinking of HL as "hearing loss."

Table 2–1. Table to convert audiogram HLs to MAF SPLs (HLs minus SPLs), the latter suitable for comparing audiogram values to free-field speech SPLs. The conversions are derived from the ISO (1961) MAF normal binaural thresholds in SPLs, modified for monaural listening by adding 3 dB to the ISO thresholds.

Frequency (in Hz)	SPL − HL (in dB)
125	24
250	14
500	9
1000	7
1500	6
2000	4
3000	0
4000	−1
6000	7.5
8000	10.5

References

American National Standard ANSI S3.20-1973. (1973). *Psychoacoustical terminology* (pp. 19, 30.) New York: Acoustical Society of America.

American Standard Practice C16.5-1954. (1961). *Volume measurements of electrical speech and program waves.* American Standards Association (now American National Standards Institute).

ISO Recommendation R 226. (1961). *Normal equal-loudness contours for pure tones and normal threshold of hearing under free field listening conditions.* International Organization for Standardization.

ISO Recommendation R 369 (1964). *Standard reference zero for the calibration of pure-tone audiometers.* International Organization for Standardization.

Killion, M. C. (1978). Revised estimate of minimum audible pressure: Where is the "missing 6 dB"? *Journal of the Acoustical Society of America, 63,* 1501–1508.

Shaw, E. A. G. (1974). The external ear. In W. D. Keidel & W. D. Neff (Eds.), *Handbook of sensory physiology* (pp. 455–490). Berlin: Springer-Verlag.

Sivian, L. J., & White, S. D. (1933). On mimimum audible sound fields. *Journal of the Acoustical Society of America, 4,* 288–321.

Villchur, E. (1957). *Handbook of sound reproduction* (p. 8). Mineola, NY: Radio Magazines.

Villchur, E. (1965). *Reproduction of sound* (p. 6). New York: Dover Publications.

CHAPTER 3

Acoustic Resonators

RESONANCE

A vibrating source of sound free of external control, such as a tuning fork or a plucked guitar string, continuously interchanges energy between its elastic and inertial-mass elements. At the point of maximum displacement the vibrating mass has come to momentary rest before reversing its motion, and the mass has zero kinetic energy. Potential energy stored in the elastic element, which at this point is strained the most, is at a maximum. When the mass element returns to its original position of zero displacement there is no tension on the spring at all, but the mass has reached its highest velocity and its kinetic energy is at maximum. The values of mass and elasticity determine the frequency of this interchange of energy, just as the values of inductance and capacitance in a tuned electrical circuit determine the rate of interchange of electrical energy between coil and capacitor. The frequency of the interchange of energy is called the *resonance frequency*.[1]

---

[1]Use of the term "resonant frequency" for "resonance frequency" is fairly common (including in my own writing of 30 years ago), but as the late Professor Frederick Hunt was fond of pointing out, a frequency cannot be resonant. One may refer to a resonant device or to its resonance frequency, which is to say its frequency of resonance.

Friction, mechanical or acoustical, *damps* the vibration in the same way that electrical resistance damps an electrical oscillation, by absorbing and finally using up all of the energy. Without damping, the vibration would go on forever without any further addition of energy, because the mass and elastic elements of a resonant system can only store energy temporarily, not absorb it.

The resonance frequency of a mass-elasticity system is reduced as the mass is increased or the elastic stiffness is decreased, according to a relatively simple relationship:

$$f = \frac{1}{2\pi\sqrt{MC}}$$

where f = resonance frequency

M = mass of the inertial element

C = compliance of the elastic element

This equation explains why the low-frequency strings of a piano or violin are heavier, and why tightening the strings raises their resonance frequencies.

The basic elements of a resonant system are inertia and restoring force or their analogs. In the examples above these elements are supplied by mass and elasticity, but the functions of inertia and restoring force can also be supplied by electrical inductance and capacitance, and gravity rather than elasticity may supply restoring force (in the resonant system of a pendulum, for example, or of water sloshing back and forth in a bowl). Increasing either the mass of a pendulum or the length of its arm reduces its resonance frequency.

If a mechanical or acoustical system with mass and elasticity is stimulated without being subjected to control it will vibrate at its own natural resonance frequency. When such a system is subjected to forced vibration, however, it must vibrate at the frequency of the stimulus. The amplitude of the enforced vibration, which is the system's response, increases as the frequency of the stimulus approaches the resonance frequency of the system, with maximum response at resonance. A transmission path for sound may include elements that form acoustical resonators at one or more resonance frequencies; the external ear and ear canal or the tubing between a hearing aid and the end of an earmold are examples. Such a path will be a better conduit for sounds whose frequencies are the same as or close to one of the resonance frequencies of the path than it will for sound at other frequencies, and the transmission path will have peaks in its frequency response. *Damping*, which is to say the introduction of mechanical or acoustical friction (the electrical equivalent is *resistance*), not only prevents a resonant system from vibrating forever but reduces the response peaks in a forced-vibration system.

Two types of acoustic resonators form part of the design of current hearing aids: Helmholtz and air-column.

The Helmholtz Resonator

In the nineteenth century Hermann Helmholtz built a device that could separate a particular frequency component from a complex sound. When the enclosure illustrated in Figure 3–1A is stimulated by a complex sound at the large opening, it responds to only one frequency component of the sound, the component at the resonance frequency of the enclosure. Signal components at other frequencies are substantially prevented from getting through to the opposite opening; the

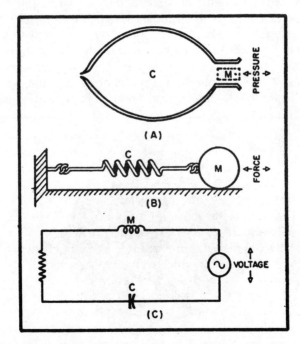

Figure 3–1. A. The Helmholtz resonator: M is the acoustic mass, or inertance, and C is the acoustic compliance. **B** and **C** are mechanical and electrical analogs of the Helmholtz resonator. (From *Handbook of Sound Reproduction*, by E. Villchur, 1957, p. 26. Mineola, New York: Radio Magazines. Reprinted with permission.)

enclosure has a single-frequency response. Figure 3–2 is the original illustration of this resonator from Helmholtz's "On the Sensations of Tone" (1954/1885). Helmholtz listened at the smaller opening, which closed it off, and applied input sound to the acoustic mass (shown in dotted lines in Figure 3–1) of the larger opening, but in most modern applications of the Helmholtz resonator the sound stimulus is applied to the elastic element, and a single opening that provides the acoustic mass serves as the output.

For an acoustical resonator to exhibit Helmholtz resonance, the dimensions of the enclosure must be small compared to the wavelength of the stimulating sound. The longest acoustical path within the enclosure is then only a small fraction of the wavelength of the input sound, so that the phase and the internal pressure state of the air at any instant will not vary significantly from one point to another. The air in the enclosure is thus compressed and rarified almost uniformly by a sound stimulus, like a pillow of air being squeezed on all sides.

The resonant elements of a Helmholtz resonator, like those of a mechanical resonator, are mass and elasticity. The elastic element is the body of enclosed air (whose elastic property is referred to as *acoustic compliance* or its reciprocal, *acoustic stiffness*), and the air in the opening to the outside supplies the mass element (called *acoustic mass* or *inertance*). These two elements form a resonant system analogous to the weight and spring or to the electrical circuit of Figure 3–1B and 3–1C.

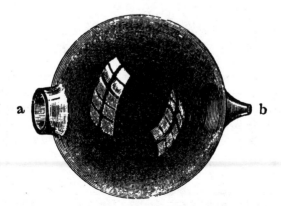

Figure 3–2. Helmholtz' drawing of the Helmholtz resonator. (From *On the Sensations of Tone*, by H. Helmholtz, 1954 reprint, p, 43. [Originally published in English translation 1885]. New York: Dover Publications. Reprinted with permission.)

What does this have to do with hearing aids? When an earmold or ITE hearing aid is vented, a Helmholtz resonator is formed by the elasticity of the air trapped in the ear canal and the acoustic mass of the air in the vent. The typical design of a vented hearing aid or earmold creates a relatively broad Helmholtz resonance in the frequency region of a few hundred Hz, which increases the output of the hearing aid in that frequency region (by an amount that depends on the degree of damping) and decreases the output below the frequency of the resonance peak.

As in any mass-elasticity system, the resonance frequency of this system is determined by the compliance of the elastic element and by the mass. The same equation presented earlier for mechanical resonance applies here: The greater the compliance and the greater the mass, the lower the resonance frequency. Thus the greater the volume of air left in the canal, and the greater the acoustic mass in the vent, the lower the resonance frequency. The acoustic mass of the air in the vent increases as the length of the vent is increased and the diameter of the vent is decreased, so that reducing the diameter of the vent with an insert lowers the resonance frequency. A deep earmold insertion leaves a smaller volume of air in the canal and raises the resonance frequency.

The Helmholtz resonance of a hearing aid is relatively broad (it does not have a sharp response peak at its resonance frequency) because the resonator is damped: it includes an element of acoustic resistance or friction. A narrow tube inserted into the vent not only reduces the resonance frequency by increasing the acoustic mass but also increases the acoustic friction between air molecules, which reduces the height of the low-frequency resonance peak.

The resonance frequency of a Helmholtz resonator depends on the volume of air in the enclosure, not its shape, a principle that can be demonstrated by a simple experiment. Blowing across the top of a bottle produces the familiar foghorn sound of its Helmholtz tone. If the bottle is partially filled with water its volume is decreased and the frequency of the tone goes up. Since the surface of the water forms one side of the enclosure, tilting the bottle will change the enclosure shape without changing its volume, and if we blow across the top of the tilted bottle we will produce a Helmholtz tone of the same frequency as for the upright bottle. Thus the Helmholtz resonance of the earcanal cavity between the end of the hearing aid and the eardrum is affected by the volume but not the shape of the cavity.

A Helmholtz resonator does not respond to stimuli at frequencies outside of its resonance-frequency region. Higher frequency sound from the hearing aid does not excite the Helmholtz resonance of cavity and vent.

The sound of a stimulated Helmholtz resonator is considered musically uninteresting, like the output of a sine-wave signal generator, and it is not often used as the basic resonator in musical wind instruments. It is used in the ocarina or "sweet potato" illustrated in Figure 3–3, and Helmholtz resonators have been used to reinforce the fundamental frequency components of low-frequency organ pipes. The Helmholtz resonance of the air and f-holes in the body of a guitar or viol instrument contributes a broad low-frequency component to the sound of the instrument.

Air-Column Resonance

Air-column resonance differs from Helmholtz resonance in that the air oscillates only along the length of the column, and at a given instant the pressure state of the air along the column varies from one point to another. The air can pulsate longitudinally at multiples of the funda-

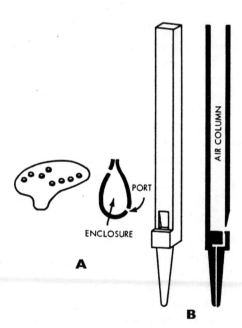

Figure 3–3. Helmholtz and air-column resonance in the ocarina and organ pipe. (From *Reproduction of Sound*, by E. Villchur, 1965, p. 8. New York: Dover Publications. Reprinted with permission.)

mental resonance frequency at the same time as at the fundamental, because it can pulsate simultaneously in sections and as a whole. When the stimulating sound includes a broad spectrum of frequency components, therefore, the oscillation of the resonator is rich in harmonic overtones, and this makes the air column suitable for musical wind instruments. An air column is the resonating element in the organ pipe of Figure 3–3.

Air-column resonance is dependent on what are called *standing waves*. A sound wave traveling along a pipe will be reflected at the end of the pipe whether the end is open or closed, because in either case the sound encounters a medium of changed impedance. When the reflected compression front of a sound wave in the pipe meets the compression front of a succeeding wave traveling toward it, the two reinforce each other; when a reflected compression front meets a rarefaction front, they cancel each other. Standing waves are formed in a pipe when the points of reinforcement and cancellation occur at fixed places along the pipe; this happens when there is a particular relation between the wavelength of the stimulating sound (determined by its frequency) and the length of the pipe. In a pipe open at one end, standing waves are formed when the the length of the pipe is a quarter of the wavelength of the stimulating sound or an odd multiple of a quarter wavelength. In a closed pipe, standing waves are formed when the length of the pipe is a half wavelength of the stimulating sound or any multiple, odd or even, of a half wavelength. The reason for the different mode of operation of open and closed pipes is that a reflection of sound from the open end of a pipe reverses the phase of the wave, and this reflection matches and reinforces the pressure state of a wave traveling in the opposite direction at a quarter-wavelength rather than a half-wavelength distance.[2]

It follows that the first air-column resonance frequency of a pipe open at one end occurs when the length of the pipe is a quarter wavelength of the stimulating sound, while the first resonance frequency of a closed-end pipe occurs when the pipe is a half wavelength of the

---

[2]A compression front will be reflected from the open end of a pipe as a rarefaction front; it will travel back and reach the closed end of a quarter-wavelength pipe two quarter-wavelength trips after the compression front left the closed end. This is half a cycle after the compression front was generated; the original signal will have advanced half a cycle to its rarefaction phase, and it meets the reflected rarefaction front in phase. For a closed pipe, a compression front will be reflected as a compression front, and it will reach the other end of a half-wavelength pipe two half-wavelength trips (one full cycle) after it left there. The original compression front will have advanced a full cycle and is in its compression phase again, so it meets the reflected compression front in phase.

stimulating sound. The effective length of an open column is increased (the frequency of resonance is lowered) by an *end correction* and by a flange at the end of the column. For the open, flanged air column of an unaided ear canal, the net effect of the end correction, combined with interaction with the concha (the latter raises the resonance frequency) is to lower the resonance frequency of the canal relative to its length by about 25%, to an average value of about 2.7 kHz.

The molecules in an air column with standing waves oscillate most vigorously (there is maximum back-and-forth velocity of the air) at points called *velocity loops*, or *velocity antinodes*, and oscillates least vigorously at points called *velocity nodes*.

Air-column resonance has significance for hearing aids in two ways. The first is that the ear canal is a resonant air column open at one end that affects the normal unaided sound at the eardrum, as shown in curve 5 of Figure 5–1 in Chapter 5. An earmold or ITE hearing aid closes off the canal so that it is resonant when its effective length is a quarter wavelength rather than a half wavelength of the stimulating sound, and it also shortens the air column. These changes influence the effective frequency response of the hearing aid, as discussed in Chapter 5.

The second effect of air-column resonance on hearing aids is in the acoustic path within the hearing aid, especially in the tubing between a behind-the-ear (BTE) hearing aid and the end of the earmold. The tubing has standing-wave resonances and creates peaks in the frequency response of the hearing aid, like those shown in the top curve of Figure 3–4.

These peaks and valleys in frequency response can be smoothed out by damping elements that introduce acoustical friction into the transmission path of the sound. The damping elements are in the form of calibrated inserts, available commercially in different values of acoustical ohms. But a damping element inserted at a velocity node, where there is little activity of the air molecules, won't do much good: substantial motion of the air molecules is needed if the acoustical friction is to be effective in slowing down the oscillation. The damper must therefore be inserted at or near a velocity loop, where standing waves have created maximum longitudinal vibration of the air molecules.

Figure 3–4, from a study by Killion (1981), shows the effects of different values of damping elements on the frequency response of a BTE hearing aid, and the appropriate places to insert these elements in the resonant air column. A damper at the end of the hook, for example, is positioned closest to the loop for the fundamental resonance frequency of the tube, and reduces only the lowest frequency peak. Higher frequency peaks are created by standing waves at odd har-

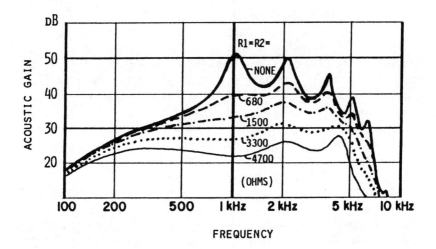

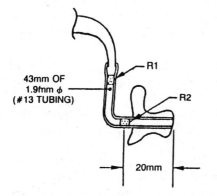

43mm OF
1.9tmm φ
(#13 TUBING)

Figure 3–4. Effect of damping inserts on the frequency response of a BTE hearing aid. (From "Earmold Options for Wideband Hearing Aids," by M. C. Killion, 1981, p. 12. *Journal of Speech and Hearing Disorders, 46.* Reprinted with permission.)

monics of the fundamental resonance frequency and need to be damped at the loop positions of these standing waves. (The second peak in Figure 3–4, which seems to be at an even harmonic of the fundamental, is created by a resonance in the hearing aid rather than in the tubing.) The damper in Figure 3–4 at the midpoint of the tubing is a compromise position that smooths out the higher frequency peaks.

Dampers may become clogged with moisture, but dampers in the hook have better protection against moisture. Some manufacturers place dampers in the hook—either a damper near the tip or a damper at each end—to serve as the total damping system.

In the field of sound reproduction the benefit of avoiding peaks in the frequency response of reproducing equipment is accepted as obvious: Smooth response produces a more natural sound for both music and speech. This is also true of hearing aids, but in hearing aids there are additional and potentially more important disadvantages to response peaks. The first is that a hearing-impaired person with recruitment (see Chapter 6) hears a change of sound intensity with an exaggerated contrast in loudness; such a listener may hear an 8-dB amplitude peak the way a normal listener hears a peak of 16 dB or more. Sound that contains appreciable energy at the frequency of a large peak in hearing-aid response often causes discomfort, and a person wearing peaky hearing aids will tend to set the volume controls at levels lower than optimum to avoid intermittent discomfort from signals that appear in the frequency region of the peak or peaks.

This effect of response peaks may be critical in cases of profound deafness, in which the dynamic range of residual hearing is typically reduced severely by recruitment. In Figure 3–5 the frequency response of the undamped BTE hearing aid shown in Figure 3–4 is plotted against the average dynamic/frequency range of hearing, between threshold and discomfort, of a group of profoundly deaf children (the latter data measured by Boothroyd, 1974). The peak in hearing-aid response at 1 kHz would prevent a listener with the dynamic range of

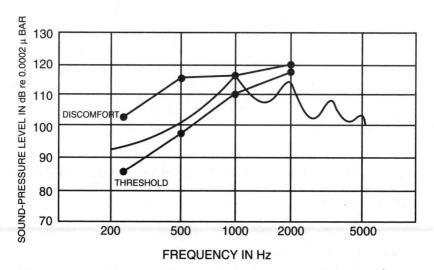

Figure 3–5. Frequency response of the undamped BTE hearing aid from Figure 3–4, plotted against the average dynamic range of hearing, between threshold and discomfort, of a group of profoundly deaf children. The response peak at 1 kHz prevents the impaired listener from using most of his or her severely restricted residual dynamic range of hearing without accepting discomfort from signals in the 1 kHz region. A damper at the end of the hook is needed.

hearing of Figure 3–5 from using more overall gain than that shown in the diagram: At higher gain, signal components in the frequency region of the peak would be amplified past the listener's discomfort level from time to time. A large part of the residual hearing shown in Figure 3–5 remains unused because the gain of the hearing aid has to be set low enough to avoid discomfort from signals in one narrow frequency region. A damper at the end of the hook would bring down or eliminate the 1-kHz peak, would allow a higher gain setting, and would make the hearing aid much more effective for this listener.

A second damaging effect of frequency-response peaks in hearing aids is that peaks allow acoustic feedback to occur at lower overall levels. The gain of the hearing aid is, of course, greatest at the frequency of the peak or peaks, and that is where the feedback takes off. Acoustic feedback depends on two things: the amount of gain at the frequency of the whistle, and the leakage of sound from the output of the hearing-aid receiver back to the microphone input. Reducing a frequency-response peak in a hearing aid by 6 dB will allow the overall gain to be increased by 6 dB before feedback occurs, assuming there are no other intermediate peaks.

Acoustical resonance is integral both to the operation of the unaided ear and to the combined system of ear and hearing aid.

References

Boothroyd. A. (1974). Sensory capabilities in normal and hearing-impaired children. In R. E. Stark (Ed.), *Sensory capabilities of hearing-impaired children* (p. 42). Baltimore: University Park Press; also personal communication.

Helmholtz, H. (1954). *On the sensations of tone* (p. 43) [Original English translation 1885]. New York: Dover Publications.

Killion, M. C. (1981). Earmold options for wideband hearing aids. *Journal of Speech and Hearing Disorders, 46,* 10–20.

Villchur, E. (1957). *Handbook of sound reproduction* (p. 26). Mineola, NY: Radio Magazines.

Villchur, E. (1965). *Reproduction of sound* (p. 8). New York: Dover Publications.

CHAPTER 4

Horns

The horn is an ancient acoustic device, whose principle is used in as simple a procedure as putting a cupped hand to the ear for listening or to the mouth for shouting. It is commonly used to give musical instruments or the human voice a better bite of the air, enabling them to produce sound of greater intensity. What a horn does *not* do is "amplify" the sound. The process of amplification, in its engineering sense, requires that additional power be injected into a system so that the output power is greater than the input power. A horn merely increases a system's efficiency in using a given input power.

The human voice has relatively poor coupling to the air into which it radiates. The intensity of the sound we can produce is limited more by the inefficient engagement of air by our voice mechanisms than by the power of our lungs. A horn such as a megaphone allows the voice mechanism of the speaker to engage the air more efficiently and to radiate more of the speaker's potential sound power. The horn does this by providing the speaker with the equivalent of a large radiating diaphragm.

The air in the horn shown in Figure 4–1 may be thought of as a succession of imaginary, infinitesimally thin cross-sectional layers. A vibrating body at the narrow end, or *throat*, is in immediate contact with the first of these layers and will progressively engage each of the succeeding layers of air confined by the walls of the horn. Because the increase in area from one layer to the next is very small (the "imped-ance discontinuity" between layers is small), very little energy is lost

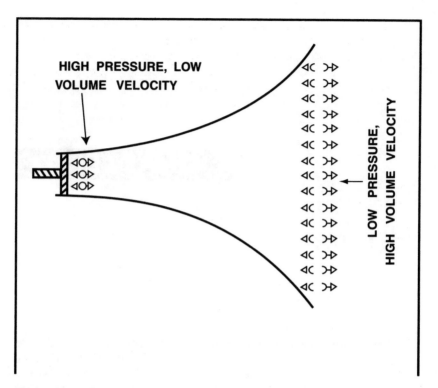

Figure 4–1. The horn as an impedance-matching device. The SPL at the mouth is greater than the original SPL at the throat (without the presence of the horn), by an amount equal to the acoustic gain of the horn. (After *Reproduction of Sound,* by E. Villchur, 1957, p. 110. Mineola, NY: Radio Magazines.)

in the transfer. The horn has an almost massless virtual diaphragm at its large end, or *mouth,* coupled to the source of sound at the throat by the intervening layers of air; the molecules of air at the mouth of the horn vibrate back and forth as if a diaphragm the size of the mouth were there. The effective radiating area of the actual diaphragm at the throat is increased to the approximate area of the mouth.

Although the horn contributes no new power to a system, when an acoustic-power generator is inefficiently coupled to its load the horn allows more power to be drawn from the generator: The power radiated from the horn's mouth is increased by an amount equal to the increase in area from the throat to the mouth of the horn, assuming the generator has the required power capacity. Because sound pressure varies as the square root of the acoustic power in a given medium, the SPL at the mouth of the horn is increased as the square root of the increase in area. If the area from throat to mouth is quadrupled the the sound pressure is doubled, the power is quadrupled, and the acoustic gain of the horn in either pressure or power is 6 dB.

In engineering terms a horn is an acoustic impedance-matching device, analogous to an electric transformer or a mechanical lever. The horn shown in Figure 4–1 acts as a bridge between a high-impedance source at the throat and a low-impedance load at the mouth.[1] The horn reflects a load back to the diaphragm that enables the diaphragm to work harder, just as the blades of an electric fan make it possible for the shaft to engage more air. The small diaphragm in Figure 4–1, by itself, could be driven by a locomotive engine without improving its ability to radiate acoustic power.

In Figure 4–1 the sound travels from the throat to the mouth, from high impedance to low impedance, but the horn will perform the same impedance-matching function going the other way, from mouth to throat, as in acoustic hearing aids. A horn will increase the efficiency of the transfer of energy from a high-impedance source to a low-impedance load, or from a low-impedance source to a high-impedance load.

HORN DESIGN

Three characteristics of horns that relate directly to hearing aids are the amount of increase of area from throat to mouth, the area of the mouth, and the rate of flare.

The greater the increase of area from the throat to the mouth of a horn, the greater the acoustic load reflected back to a source of sound at the throat and the greater the acoustic gain of the horn. The greater the absolute area of the mouth, the larger the virtual diaphragm and the more power the horn can radiate. But there are clearly practical limits to the mouth area, and the allowable area of the mouth is also affected by the rate of flare between the throat and mouth. The rate of flare determines what is called the *cutoff frequency*; below this frequency the loading effect of the horn drops off quickly and the horn disap-

[1]The sound pressure at the throat of the horn in Figure 4–1 is high relative to sound pressure at the mouth, while the air molecules at the throat have low velocity relative to velocity at the mouth. But the horn, by increasing the load on the acoustic generator, allows the generator to develop a higher SPL at the throat. The sound pressure at the mouth is less than the pressure at the throat, but because the throat pressure has been increased, the pressure at the mouth still exceeds the original sound pressure of the generator (less horn) by the amount of acoustic gain.

pears acoustically. The faster the flare, the higher the cutoff frequency; it follows that the rate of flare must be kept low to avoid too high a cutoff frequency. A slow flare rate combined with a large mouth area adds up to a long horn. This explains the many coils of an instrument like the tuba: the mouth of the tuba must be large in order to make a lot of sound by engaging a large volume of air, but the rate of flare must be kept low for the horn to be capable of operating down to very low frequencies. It takes 18 feet of coiled brass to get from the small-diameter mouthpiece to the large bell-shaped mouth.

HORNS IN ACOUSTIC HEARING AIDS

Horns used as acoustic hearing aids, such as those in Figure 4–2 (from a 1902 Sears Roebuck catalog), increased the efficiency of the transfer of energy from the air to the ear canal, thus working from the mouth of the horn to its throat and matching a low-impedance source to a higher impedance load. The larger the mouth of such a hearing aid, the greater the increase in sound pressure it was able to produce at its narrow throat; but too fast a rate of flare had to be avoided to keep the cutoff frequency low enough to be effective for speech. It was therefore necessary to combine a slow rate of flare with as large a mouth as was acceptable, which explains the considerable length of the hearing-aid tube in Figure 4–2, and the internal design of the Sears "London Hearing Horn" shown in Figure 4–3. The "London" horn is folded back on itself twice, tripling the length of its acoustic path without increasing the size of the device. The longer path allowed a reduced rate of flare, lowering the cutoff frequency and extending the effectiveness of the horn to lower frequencies. This internal folding was reinvented almost half a century later for use in public-address loudspeakers, and is known today as the re-entrant horn.

Hearing tubes like the one in Figure 4–2 had one advantage over most modern hearing aids: the speaker could talk right into the mouthpiece, which created a greatly improved signal-to-noise ratio. As horns, these tubes typically provided a sound-pressure gain of the order of 10 dB at speech frequencies, but when advantage was taken of their close-talking feature very high ear canal SPLs could be achieved. As in the case of the re-entrant horn that adapted an old design, this close-talking feature has been adapted to modern use; some hearing-aid systems place the microphone at the talker rather than the listener position (e.g., in classrooms).

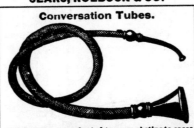

These Tubes are adapted to more obstinate cases of deafness, are very finely constructed throughout, lined with a peculiar spiral wire, which, although admitting of great flexibility, keeps the tube fully distended in any position.

No. 20R410 Conversation Tube, 3 feet in length, fine quality flexible mohair, hard rubber ends. Price ....(If by mail, postage extra, 8c) . .$1.40

No. 20R412 Conversation Tube, highest grade, flexible mohair, tapered tube, 3 feet in length, hard rubber mountings. Suitable for the most obstinate cases of deafness. Price.................$1.65
  If by mail, postage extra, 15 cents.

No. 20R414 Conversation Tube. Same size and style as No. 20R412 but covered with best grade black silk. Price....................................$1.89
  If by mail, postage extra, 15 cents.

Hearing Horns.

These horns are exactly the same as those advertised by many dealers at prices ranging from $8.00 to $15.00 each. These London Hearing Horns are constructed of light metal upon an entirely new principle. They may be carried in the pocket and when in use are easily concealed in the hand. They are designed for the use of those who are only moderately deaf and enable one to hear not only an ordinary conversation but sounds at a distance as well, making them suitable for use anywhere—at home, in church, or public entertainments.

Made in Two Sizes, with Black Oxidized Finish.

No. 20R420 London Hearing Horn, medium size. 2½ inches in length. Price, each.................$1.29
  If by mail, postage extra, 5 cents.

No. 20R421 London Hearing Horn, large size, 4 inches in length. Price, each....................$1.35
  If by mail, postage extra, 8 cents.

Your money will be promptly refunded if the horn does not give entire satisfaction.

Figure 4–2. Acoustic hearing aids, from a Sears, Roebuck catalog of 1902.

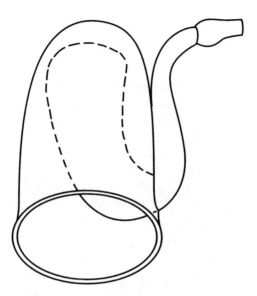

Figure 4–3. Construction of the "London hearing horn" shown in Figure 4–2. The folded design triples the length of the horn without increasing the size of the device.

HORNS IN MODERN HEARING AIDS

Far more often than not, hearing aids require high-frequency emphasis. Mead Killion has designed a system of tubing between a BTE hearing aid and the inner tip of the earmold[2] that can provide 6 dB or more of high-frequency emphasis. The tubing incorporates a horn whose rate of flare is chosen to provide a midrange cutoff frequency; the cutoff slope of the horn provides the rising part of the high-frequency response of the hearing aid. Killion gives the approximate cutoff frequency in kHz as 117 divided by the average distance in millimeters over which the diameter doubles.

Figure 4–4, from Killion (1981), shows the design of this type of horn and its effect on the frequency response of the hearing aid. In this illustration the diameter of the mouth of the horn exhausting into the ear canal is something less than double the diameter of the throat (four times the area); at double the diameter the sound pressure would be doubled, and there would be 6 dB extra output above the

[2]Killion cites the work of Sam Lybarger, who had previously described dual-diameter transmission paths for hearing aids.

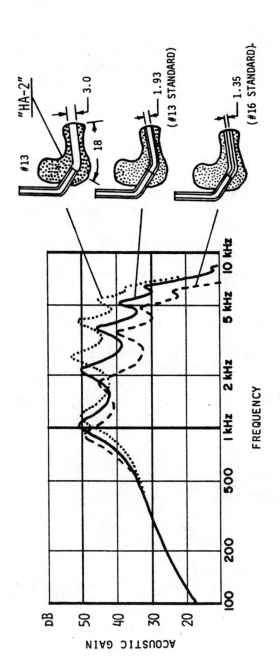

Figure 4—4. The Killion horn (top) in the tubing of a BTE hearing aid. If the diameter of the throat, the horn provides 6 dB additional acoustic output above the cutoff frequency. (From "Earmold Options for Wideband Hearing Aids," by M. C. Killion, 1981, p. 12. *Journal of Speech and Hearing Disorders, 46.* Reprinted with permission.)

cutoff frequency. If the distance over which the diameter doubles is 43 mm, the cutoff frequency (117/43) is 2.7 kHz. Sound pressure above the cutoff frequency is doubled, and sound pressure below the cutoff frequency drops off to its low-frequency value in about an octave. The low-frequency sound pressure is unaffected by the horn.

The horn shown in Figure 4–4 is made up of discrete sections of successively greater diameter. A molded, one-section horn is far more convenient than a horn made of sections glued together by the audiologist. Such a horn was designed by Libby (1982), and is commercially available.

The Killion horn provides 6 dB of high-frequency gain free, in the sense that for a given amplifier/receiver it gives the hearing aid 6 dB more of high-frequency acoustical output. The horn design taps into a high-frequency power capability that was unused. This has an obvious advantage for hearing aids that do not provide the high-frequency emphasis needed for a particular patient, and it has a vital advantage in cases of severe to profound deafness in which the hearing aid does not have enough high-frequency power or begins to distort at the necessary power.

ANSI Standard S3.22-1996 recommends use of either the HA-2 or HA-4 coupler for measuring BTE hearing aids. The HA-2 provides a stepped-diameter entrance to the coupler cavity, which approximates the horn effect of the Killion design. It is the coupler to use for a BTE hearing aid that will be used with horn tubing. If a different coupler is used for such a hearing aid, the measurement should be made through the horn tubing and earmold of the aid. When an HA-2 coupler is used to measure a hearing aid that will be used with constant-diameter tubing, the horn effect of the coupler must be subtracted from the coupler curve.

References

American National Standard S3.22-1996. (1996). *Specification of hearing aid characteristics* (p. 5). New York: Acoustical Society of America.

Killion, M. C. (1981). Earmold options for wideband hearing aids. *Journal of Speech and Hearing Disorders, 46,* 10–20.

Libby, E. R. (1982). In search of transparent insertion gain hearing aid responses. In Studebaker & Bess (Ed.), *The Vanderbilt hearing-aid report* (pp. 112–123). Upper Darby: Monographs in Contemporary Audiology.

The Sears, Roebuck Catalogue. (1902). 1969 reprint. New York: Bounty Books.

Villchur, E. (1957). *Handbook of Sound Reproduction* (p. 110). Mineola, NY: Radio Magazines.

CHAPTER 5

The Acoustical Transmission Path of the Ear

The frequency response of an electronic amplifier can be defined simply: It is the relative amplitude of output signals at different frequencies, under normal conditions of amplifier use,[1] when the amplifier input is swept by a flat signal. The operating frequency response of a hearing aid, however, has a more complex definition. Flat electrical and acoustical frequency response of the hearing aid itself, even when working into an appropriate cavity, does not provide flat frequency response for the hearing aid in the ear. That is because the physical presence of a hearing aid or earmold changes the natural frequency response of the unaided ear's transmission path.

An amplifier is considered electrically transparent if it can be inserted into a system without creating any audible changes other than increased output. For a hearing aid to be acoustically transparent, the sound pressures it produces at the eardrum in response to external sound stimuli at different frequencies must not differ, outside of

[1]Conditions of amplifier use that affect frequency response include the operating power level and the output load.

increased amplitude, from those that would be produced by the same stimuli with the hearing aid removed. In terms of frequency response, an acoustically transparent hearing aid is said to have flat *insertion gain*. The insertion gain of a hearing aid is the difference between the aided and unaided gain of the ear over the frequency spectrum: It is the combined gain of the hearing aid and occluded ear (the latter gain changed by the presence of the aid or earmold) minus the gain of the open, unaided ear.

EFFECTS OF THE EXTERNAL EAR ON THE EFFECTIVE FREQUENCY RESPONSE OF A HEARING AID

An unaided ear does not have flat frequency response; sound pressures at the eardrum are affected differently at different frequencies by the acoustical transmission path of the ear. The insertion of an earmold or hearing aid into the ear canal changes the normal frequency response of the unemcumbered transmission path, and these changes must be counted as part of the frequency response of the hearing aid. Variations in eardrum sound pressure introduced by the physical presence of the hearing aid are just as meaningful as variations in the frequency response of the hearing aid itself. The same principle operates in electronic circuits; when we insert a new component into a circuit, we must consider not only the frequency response of the component but its possible effect on the frequency response of the rest of the circuit.

Pioneering studies of the acoustics of the external ear were made by E. A. G. Shaw. Figure 5–1, from Shaw (1974), shows the acoustic gain in an average ear,[2] from free field to eardrum, of different parts of the unaided transmission path. Each element of the path can be changed by a hearing aid, but hearing aids of different types affect different elements, depending on the physical design of the aid, how it is worn, and the location of the microphone. The diffraction effects of the head (curve 1) and reflections from the torso and neck (curve 2) are changed by hearing aids worn on the body; the effect of the pinna flange (curve 4) is changed when the microphone is located outside the external ear, as in behind-the-ear (BTE) hearing aids; in-the-ear (ITE) hearing aids or the earmolds of behind-the-ear aids change ear-

[2]Wiener and Ross (1946) reported that the characteristics of ear-transmission paths for individual subjects varied from the average by a standard deviation of 1 dB or less below 500 Hz, about 3 dB at 5 kHz, and 5 dB or more above 5 kHz.

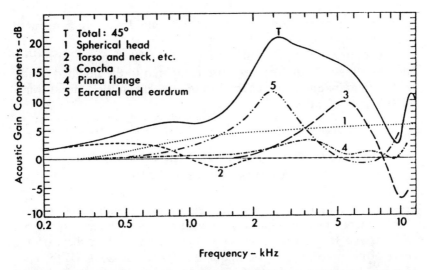

Figure 5–1. Acoustic gain, from free field to eardrum, of different parts of the transmission path of an average ear. Azimuth of sound is 45°. The overall gain at 0° (the listener facing the source of sound) is about 5 dB less than at 45°; gain at other azimuths is also less. "Total" curve represents addition of parts in the order shown. (From "The External Ear," by E. A. G. Shaw, 1974, p. 468. In W. D. Keidel & W. D. Neff [Eds.], *Handbook of Sensory Physiology.* Berlin: Springer-Verlag. Reprinted with permission.)

canal resonance (curve 5) by closing off and shortening the canal air column, and they normally fill the concha and bypass its acoustical effect (curve 3); completely-in-the-canal (CIC) hearing aids also change ear-canal resonance but do not fill the concha.

The most significant change in the acoustical transmission path of the ear caused by the presence of a hearing aid is the change in resonance frequency of the ear canal. Curve 5 of Figure 5–1 shows a peak at about 2.5 kHz, created by the air-column resonance of the ear canal as terminated at one end by the eardrum and at the other end by a flanged opening, and curve T shows the peak shifted to about 2.7 kHz because of interaction between the canal and the concha. When a hearing aid or earmold is placed in the ear canal it has two nonelectronic effects: It shortens the resonating air column, usually by at least half, and it closes off the opening to the canal. Cutting the effective length of the ear canal by half doubles the resonance frequency. Changing from an open to a closed air column shifts the fundamental resonance mode from quarter-wave to half-wave (see Chapter 3), doubling the resonance frequency a second time; closing off the canal also eliminates the end correction and interaction with the concha. The net result is to raise the resonance frequency into the 13-kHz region, out of the frequency range of most hearing aids.

In summary, the physical presence of the hearing aid introduces effective dips in frequency response compared to the unaided condition, by eliminating some of the response peaks in the natural transmission path of the ear.

CORFIG (COUPLER RESPONSE FOR FLAT INSERTION GAIN)

The most common way to measure hearing aids is with a 2-cc coupler. The frequency-response curve produced by this coupler differs from the effective frequency response of the hearing aid in the ear (the curve of its insertion gain vs. frequency) for two reasons: (1) the coupler measurement does not take into account changes in the acoustical transmission path of the ear introduced by the hearing aid, as discussed above; and (2) the acoustical load presented to the hearing aid by a 2-cc coupler is not an accurate simulation of the load presented by an average ear.

As a result of the second factor, the 2-cc coupler measurement fails to include a real-ear increase in high-frequency response created by the increase of canal-cavity impedance presented to the hearing aid at higher frequencies. When a high-impedance generator (the hearing-aid receiver) is connected to a low-impedance load (the canal cavity), changes in the load impedance affect the amplitude of signals across the load, which is to say the output of the hearing aid. At lower frequencies the compliance of the eardrum is a significant part of the total compliance into which the hearing aid works, but as the frequency is raised the effective mass of the eardrum makes the eardrum increasingly resistant to motion. At higher frequencies, therefore, the effective volume of the canal cavity is reduced and the cavity impedance is increased, creating a rising real-ear hearing-aid response relative to its 2-cc response, as shown in Figure 5–2 (from Killion and Revit, 1993).

Fortunately the study of Killion and Revit (1993) has made it easy to include both of the effects described above in calculating the insertion-gain frequency response of a hearing aid from its 2-cc coupler measurement. Figure 5–3, from that study, is a family of "CORFIG" 2-cc coupler response curves that are corrected for these effects, and that represent flat insertion gain over the frequency spectrum for different types of hearing aids in an average ear. Each of the CORFIG curves compensates for changes to the natural frequency response of the ear

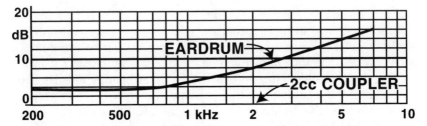

Figure 5-2. Comparison between eardrum (or Zwislocki coupler) and 2-cc sound pressure for a hearing aid or insert earphone. The rising high-frequency eardrum response reflects the progressive stiffening of the eardrum at higher frequencies, and the consequent increasing impedance of the load presented to a hearing aid. (From "CORFIG and GIFROC: Real Ear to Coupler and Back," by M. C. Killion and L. Revit, 1993. In Studebaker and Hochberg [Eds.], *Acoustical Factors Affecting Hearing-Aid performance*, p. 67. Baltimore: University Park Press. Reprinted with permission.)

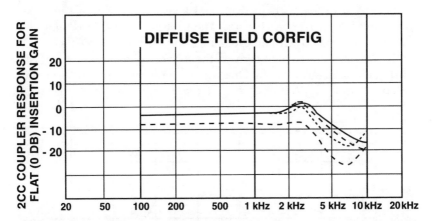

Figure 5-3. CORFIG curves: 2-cc coupler response for flat insertion gain of a hearing aid in a diffuse field. Solid line is for a BTE hearing aid; dashed line, a full-concha ITE; dotted line, a small ITC; and bottom dashed line, a deep-canal CIC. A hearing aid with flat insertion gain does not have a flat 2-cc coupler curve but one of the CORFIG curves. (From "CORFIG and GIFROC: Real Ear to Coupler and Back," by M. C. Killion and L. J. Revit, 1993. In Studebaker and Hochberg [Eds.], *Acoustical Factors Affecting Hearing-Aid Performance*, p. 79. Baltimore: University Park Press. Reprinted with permission.)

introduced by the physical presence of the hearing aid, and also compensates for the inaccurate simulation by a 2-cc coupler of the real-ear acoustical load presented to the hearing aid.

Note in Figure 5–3 that for the same insertion gain the deep-canal CIC hearing aid has the lowest coupler sound pressures of the group, and that these coupler pressures dip even lower at high frequencies. Another way of putting it is that the CIC hearing aid creates higher eardrum SPLs at given 2-cc coupler SPLs, because it is working into a smaller, and therefore higher impedance, canal cavity; and it introduces more high-frequency emphasis than other hearing aids because the rigidity of the eardrum at higher frequencies has a greater proportionate effect on the smaller cavity left by the CIC hearing aid.

An ideal hearing aid, with flat insertion gain before signal processing, will not produce a flat curve in a 2-cc coupler but one of the CORFIG curves. The difference between the coupler and CORFIG curves of a hearing aid, if any, is the frequency-response correction needed to produce flat insertion gain for that aid. After such a correction has been made, signal processing to compensate for the individual subject's impairment can be introduced without being compromised by frequency-response irregularities in the initial insertion gain. In fitting a hearing aid, the audiologist needs to know both the gain required by the patient at different frequencies and levels and the actual insertion gain provided by the hearing aid. The CORFIG corrections allow the latter to be estimated without probe-microphone measurements.

There are two ways to convert the 2-cc coupler measurement of a hearing aid to insertion gain. One way is to plot the 2-cc curve against the appropriate CORFIG curve on a graph, and then plot a curve of

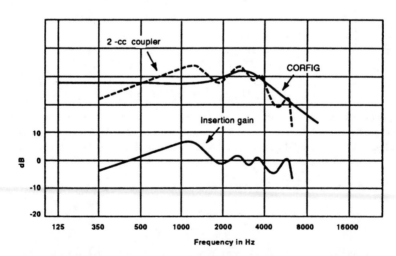

Figure 5–4. The difference between the 2-cc coupler curve (dashed line) and the CORFIG curve (upper solid line) of a BTE hearing aid is its frequency response in terms of insertion gain (lower solid line). A damper at the end of the BTE hook would reduce the frequency-response peak near 1 kHz (see Figure 3–4 in Chapter 3).

the differences, as in Figure 5–4; this curve represents the frequency response of the aid in terms of insertion gain. The other way is to use a computer-controlled fitting program called the FIG6 Hearing Aid Fitting Protocol (1987), which has the capability of factoring into its target curves the differences between 2-cc coupler response and the CORFIG curve suitable to the type of hearing aid. FIG6 calculates target frequency-response curves for a hearing aid at different input levels on the basis of the individual patient's audiogram, and these curves may be called up either directly or in the form of CORFIG-corrected curves, the latter representing target frequency responses for 2-cc coupler measurements.

Figure 5–5 shows two forms of FIG6 projections of high-level (95-dB input)[3] target-gain curves for a particular patient: the "REIG" (real-ear insertion gain) curve and the 2-cc coupler curve for a BTE hearing aid. The REIG curve represents the high-input level, real-ear frequency-response compensation calculated by FIG6 for the hearing impairment of the patient; it is the target frequency response for programming a hearing aid known to have flat insertion gain, or it is the target for probe-microphone eardrum measurements of a hearing aid whether or not the aid has flat insertion gain. A hearing aid is known to have flat insertion gain for an average ear when its coupler frequency response matches the corresponding CORFIG curve of Figure 5–3.

The FIG6 2-cc target curve incorporates the same compensation for the patient's particular hearing impairment as the REIG curve, but is also corrected for the differences between coupler and real-ear frequency response. It is the frequency-response curve we would try to match in a 2-cc measurement of the hearing aid this patient will use; it combines compensation for the subject's impairment with the CORFIG corrections. When the measured 2-cc coupler curve of the hearing aid is plotted against the FIG6 2-cc target curve, the difference between the two curves, if any, is the frequency-response compensation needed by this hearing aid for the patient whose audiogram has been entered. The imperfect simulation of the ear by the 2-cc coupler has been accounted for and is no longer a factor.

Neither of the 95-dB target curves of Figure 5–5 predicts the compensation required by the patient's impairment at lower input levels (see the discussion of recruitment and compression in Chapter 9); this compensation is plotted in the lower level (40-dB and 65-dB) target curves of FIG6, and is also calculated by FIG6 in terms of compression

[3]The frequency-response curve for 80-dB input, needed for fitting a hearing aid like the Resound, may be interpolated between the 95- and 65-db FIG6 curves.

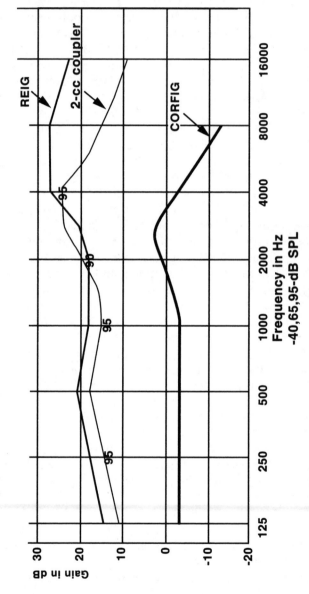

Figure 5–5. 2-cc and REIG (real-ear insertion gain) high-level (95 dB) target gains for a BTE hearing aid, projected by FIG6 fitting program on the basis of a patient's audiogram. Note that the difference between the two target gains is the CORFIG curve for BTEs. The target gain for 80-dB input may be interpolated between the 95- and 65-dB FIG6 targets.

ratios. Compression ratios and the predictable average relation between a patient's hearing impairment at threshold and at higher levels are discussed in Chapter 9.

The difference between the REIG and 2-cc curves, plotted at the bottom of the graph, is also the CORFIG curve for BTEs. The FIG6 fitting system is discussed again in Chapter 9.

The BTE CORFIG curve and the FIG6 BTE coupler correction apply to BTE hearing aids with horn tubing when the coupler measurement is made on an HA-2 coupler, which simulates horn tubing (see Chapter 4). If the HA-1 coupler normally used for ITE hearing aids is used to measure a BTE aid with either fixed-bore or horn tubing, the CORFIG and FIG6 BTE curves apply to coupler measurements made through the tubing and earmold the patient will actually use.

Hearing-aid manufacturers commonly supply BTE frequency-response curves made on an HA-2 coupler. For BTE hearing aids that use fixed-bore tubing, the horn effect must be subtracted from the HA-2 coupler curves before the latter can be compared to the CORFIG or FIG6 curves, as noted in Chapter 4.

Zwislocki (1971a,b) designed a coupler that reproduces the acoustical characteristics of an average human ear accurately. The KEMAR manikin[4] (Burkhard & Sachs, 1975) has Zwislocki couplers in its ears. With this manikin, accurate instrument measurements of hearing aids and of effects in the free field can be made. KEMAR includes simulations of pinna, ear canal, and head-diffraction effects; hearing aids can be inserted into KEMAR's mechanical ears (see Figure 5–6), or earphones can be placed over them. Killion and Revit (1993) calculated each CORFIG curve as the difference between the 2-cc coupler curve of a particular type of hearing aid and the diffuse-field frequency response of that aid mounted on KEMAR.

There are now two additional ear simulators like the Zwislocki; the IEC 711-1982 and the ANSI simulator described in ANSI Standard S3.25-1989 (1989). But whether accurate couplers, 2-cc couplers with CORFIG compensation, or probe-tube measurements are used, the electronic fitting of a hearing aid must proceed from knowledge of the real-ear insertion gain of the hearing aid.

[4]KEMAR is an acronym for Knowles Electronics Manikin for Acoustic Research.

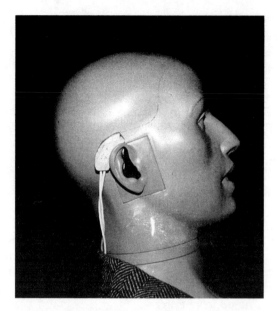

Figure 5–6. Head of the KEMAR manikin wearing a BTE hearing aid and earmold. (Courtesy of Etymotic Research.)

References

American National Standard ANSI S3.25-1989. (1989). *American National Standard for an occluded ear simulator*. New York: Acoustical Society of America.

Burkhard, M. D., & Sachs, R. M. (1975). Anthropometric manikin for acoustic research. *Journal of the Acoustical Society of America, 58,* 214–222.

FIG6. (1987). Hearing aid fitting protocol [Software and instructions]. Elk Grove Village, IL: Etymotic Research.

Killion, M. C., & Revit, L. J. (1993). CORFIG and GIFROC: Real ear to coupler and back. In Studebaker & Hochberg (Eds.), *Acoustical factors affecting hearing-aid performance* (pp. 65–85). Baltimore: University Park Press.

Shaw, E. A. G. (1974). The external ear. In W. D. Keidel & W. D. Neff (Eds.), *Handbook of sensory physiology* (pp. 455–490). Berlin: Springer-Verlag.

Wiener, F. M., & Ross, D. A. (1946). The pressure distribution in the auditory canal in a progressive sound field. *Journal of the Acoustical Society of America, 18,* 401–408.

Zwislocki, J. (1971a). Ear-like coupler for calibration of earphones. *Journal of the Acoustical Society of America, 50*(A), 110.

Zwislocki, J. (1971b). *An ear-like coupler for earphone calibration.* Special Report LSC-S-9. New York: Syracuse University.

CHAPTER 6

Psychoacoustics

Psychoacoustics refers to the perception of sound rather than its objective reality. The way we perceive sound—particularly the way we judge quantitative changes—does not have a one-to-one correspondence with the physical characteristics of the sound, but the relation between the perception and the physical reality is, within a range of variation, constant for normal listeners. Although some influences on the perception of sound cannot be categorized (a noise may appear unduly loud, for example, because of a state of anxiety on the part of the listener), there are characteristic patterns of normal human perception.

Two elements of psychoacoustics are particularly significant in audiology: masking and loudness.

MASKING

Masking is defined by the American National Standards Institute (ANSI S3.20-1973) as "the process by which the threshold of audibility for one sound is raised by the presence of another (masking) sound." Masking is thus measured by the number of decibels the threshold of hearing is raised, which makes for an unambiguous measurement, but a masking sound also reduces the loudness of sounds that are at levels above threshold.

At any given level, masking sounds have the greatest effect on the perception of sounds whose frequencies are the same as or higher

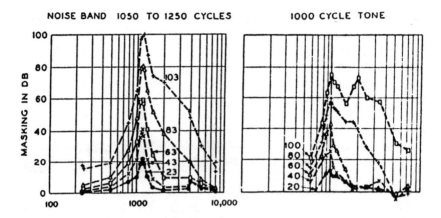

Figure 6–1. Upward spread of masking at different masker levels of a noise band and of a 1 kHz tone. The numbers on the curves are the levels of the noise or tone masker in db above hearing threshold. (From "Loudness, Its Definition, Measurement and Calculation," by H. Fletcher and W. Munson, 1933, p. 82. *Journal of the Acoustical Society of America, 9.* Reprinted with permission.)

than those of the masker. The masking of sounds whose frequencies are different from the frequency of the masker is called the *spread of masking*. Figure 6–1, from Fletcher and Munson (1937), shows the amount and spread of masking by a narrow band of noise and by a single-frequency tone. The masking effect of the tone at the masker frequency is less than that of the noise, but at higher masker levels the upward spread of masking by the tone is greater than that of the noise. For both types of maskers the relative masking of signals at frequencies higher than the masker frequency increases at higher levels.[1]

It follows from the above that the masking spread of lower frequency speech formants (see Chapter 7) will have a greater effect on higher frequency speech formants of the same vowel when the speech level is high, and that the masking spread of low-frequency noise will have a greater masking effect on higher frequency elements of speech

[1]Masking is proportionate to masker level at the masker frequency: this can be seen in Figure 6–1, where equal increases of masker levels produce equal increases of masking at the masker frequency. Allen (1997) reported that this proportionality extends over the narrow critical band of frequencies surrounding the masker frequency: that within the critical band the relative effect of masking does not change with masker level. The diagram in Figure 6–1 for pure-tone masking appears to contradict this conclusion, which Allen explains is the result of distortion products in the cochlea (personal communication).

when the noise level is raised, even though the signal-to-noise ratio does not change.

The masking of sounds that follow the masker in time is called *forward masking*. The masker has a temporary desensitizing effect on the hearing mechanism, so that for a few hundred milliseconds the threshold of hearing is raised and the loudness of sounds above threshold is reduced. A high-amplitude vowel may have this effect on a weak consonant immediately following it.

The masking of a sound that precedes the masker is called *backward masking*. Although the masker does not appear until after the signal, backward masking is possible because the listener has not completed his or her perceptive process when the signal stops. As in forward masking, backward masking may produce the masking of speech sounds by other sounds within the speech itself.

Masking is required in standard audiological testing when the impairment of one ear is significantly greater than that of the other. Test stimuli to the bad ear can elicit false responses because bone conduction through the skull sends an attenuated signal to the better ear, of the order of 50 dB lower than the stimulus in the case of supraaural earphones (depending on the coupling of the earphone to the skull), and about 70 dB lower for insert earphones. A masking signal in the opposite ear reduces that ear's sensitivity and protects against this false response. Although such masking of the opposite ear does have some small effect on the ear being tested because of central masking (masking at the cortical level), the effect is not significant: the central masking is 40–60 dB less than direct masking (Stevens & Davis, 1983). Audiometers provide narrow-band noise maskers whose center frequencies are the same as the frequency at which the subject is being tested.

LOUDNESS

The sensation of loudness is primarily associated with sound amplitude, but it is affected by other physical characteristics of the sound: its relative level, frequency, duration, and bandwidth.

Loudness Relative to Sound Pressure Level

The change of loudness with a change of sound pressure is more accurately represented by a decibel scale than by a linear scale, but the decibel scale does not reflect the relation between loudness and sound pressure very accurately either. A graph that plots the change of loudness as the sound pressure is varied is called a *loudness function*. The loudness function may be plotted in two ways. In one, a geometric loudness scale represents ratios of loudness (one point on the scale, for example, may represent double the loudness of the previous point). In the other, a linear loudness scale represents increments of loudness (each point on the scale represents a given arithmetical increase of loudness). Both forms use decibel scales for intensity, which is to say a scale that represents ratios of intensity.

Figure 6–2, from Fletcher (1938), is the more common type of loudness function, with a geometric or multiplying loudness scale. The unit of loudness on the vertical scale of Figure 6–2 is the *sone*. The sone has an absolute reference: One sone defines the loudness of a 40-phon tone (see the later section in this chapter on the phon unit), which is the same as the loudness of a 40-dB SPL tone at 1 kHz for an average unimpaired listener. The loudness in sones of any other sound is numerically equal to the ratio of its loudness to the loudness level at 40 phons: a sound twice as loud as the 40-phon reference has a loudness level of 2 sones, four times as loud as the reference, 4 sones, etc.

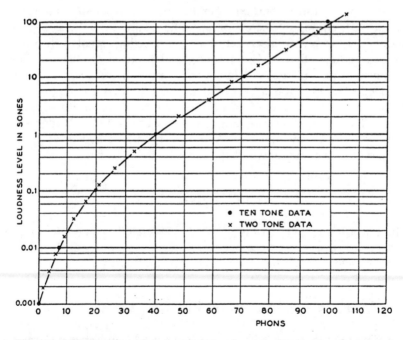

Figure 6–2. Loudness function (relation between loudness and intensity) plotted on a geometric or multiplying loudness scale. (From "Loudness, Masking, and Their Relation to the Hearing Process and the Problem of Noise Measurement," by H. Fletcher, 1938, p. 278. *Journal of the Acoustical Society of America.* Reprinted with permission.)

Above and below the 40-phon reference of the loudness scale of Figure 6–2, points are laid out at even intervals as multiples or fractions of the loudness values of previous points, although linear as well as geometric loudness scales can be calibrated in sones.[2] Figure 6–2 reflects the experimental determination that in the range above 40 phons the average normal hearing listener estimates loudness to have doubled or halved about every 10 dB of increase or decrease in sound pressure.

The units chosen for the horizontal axis of Figure 6–2 are phons rather than decibels in order to make the curve independent of frequency, but if this graph were used to represent the loudness function at 1 kHz only, the horizontal scale could be labeled dB SPL.

The second form of loudness function is shown in Figure 6–3, from Wever (1949). The loudness scale is laid out in equal increments: Each point on the scale is an addition to rather than a multiple of the loudness value of the previous point. With a linear loudness scale the loudness function is no longer the straight line above 40 phons of Figure 6–2, but a curve with a much steeper slope at high levels, which means there is a greater increase of loudness increments for a given decibel increase of SPL at high levels than for the same increase of SPL at low levels. This effect is only indirectly apparent in Figure 6–2 because the latter's geometric loudness scale has the effect built in: On the geometric scale a given increase of intensity adds more incremental units of loudness at high levels than at low levels. In any case, at high levels the audiologist can expect a greater incremental change of loudness with a given change of intensity, and more precise subject responses to such changes.

With each doubling of loudness the number of sones is also doubled. But if the sound pressure is increased in steps for equal-loudness intervals, the number of sones is increased by an equal amount for each equal increase of loudness, whatever the starting point. For

[2]The loudness in sones can be calculated for any phon level (or SPL at 1 kHz) with this slightly modified equation from Fletcher (1953):

$$\text{Loudness level in sones} = 2^{\left(\frac{\text{phons} - 40}{10}\right)}$$

The numerator of the exponent is the number of dB above or below the 40-phon reference. The number 10 in the denominator is an estimate of the sound-pressure increase in dB corresponding to a doubling of loudness (ANSI S3.20-1973), which has been changed from Fletcher's estimated value of 9. The exponent, then, is the number of times the loudness of the sound has doubled (or been cut in half) relative to the 1-sone level at 40 dB. The complete expression defines loudness level in sones as the numerical ratio of the loudness of sound at a particular phon level to the loudness of a 40-phon tone.

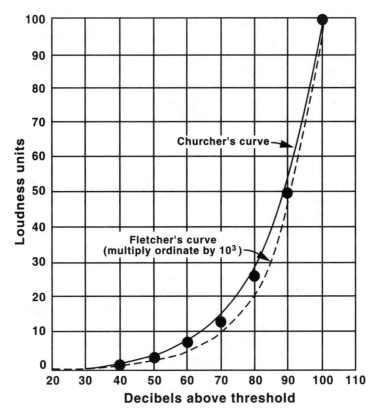

Figure 6–3. Loudness function plotted on an arithmetic or incremental loudness scale. Wever transposed the Fletcher and Churcher curves from geometric scales. The solid circles have been added to the Wever diagram: They are a plot of the equation L =kSP$^{0.6}$, where L =loudness, SP = sound pressure in μbars, and k is a constant suitable for fitting the graph to the horizontal scale. The equation is from Stevens (1955), with I$^{0.3}$ (I = intensity) converted to the equivalent SP$^{0.6}$. (From *Theory of Hearing*, by E. G. Wever, 1949, p. 301. New York: Dover Publications. Reprinted with permission.)

example, all adjacent values on the linear loudness scale of Figure 6–3, which represent increments rather than multiples, differ by the same number of sones. The entire scale represents 64 sones, and each of the 10 divisions is 6.4 sones.

Sound intensity is plotted against ratios of loudness in the geometric loudness function and against increments of loudness in the linear loudness function, but the same information can be read from either function, and either can be converted to the other. Whether a subject's loudness judgments of changing intensities produce a geometric or an incremental loudness function depends on how instructions to the subject are presented.[3] I find the scale of equal loudness increments more closely tied to subjective experience, but others take the opposite view.

Recruitment

The loudness functions shown in Figures 6–2 and 6–3 would not have much meaning for designing and fitting hearing aids if they represented the way both normal and hearing-impaired persons hear. Cochlear hearing impairment, however, typically includes a pathology called *recruitment*, which affects the way loudness changes with changes of intensity. A hearing-impaired person with recruitment has a greater hearing loss for weak sounds than for high-intensity sounds; indeed, in subjects with complete recruitment the hearing reverts to normal at some high level, so that intense sounds have the same loudness as they have for normal listeners.

Figure 6–4, from an article by Steinberg and Gardner (1937) who first analyzed recruitment, shows the effects of two forms of recruitment on the relation between loudness and sound intensity. Steinberg and Gardner used subjects with one normal and one impaired ear, and measured the relative intensities of tones presented to the normal and impaired ears at different input levels that produced the same loudness in each ear. The curves of Figure 6–4 were derived from these comparisons, but the curves may also be taken as plotting loudness (the vertical scale) against intensity (the horizontal scale). The normal loudness function is here represented by a straight 45° dashed line, an arbitrary reference that facilitates comparison with the abnormal loudness functions. The loudness functions affected by recruitment are represented by the curved lines, whose values are not absolute but calculated relative to the normal function. Figure 6–4 (left) represents what is called *complete recruitment*, and Figure 6–4 (right) *incomplete*

---

[3]If normal-hearing subjects are asked to double the loudness of a 40-dB SPL tone four times in succession, they choose levels in approximately 10-dB steps at 50, 60, 70, and 80 dB SPL. For the range between 40 dB (1 sone) and 80 dB (16 sones), this corresponds to successive increases of 1, 2, 4, and 8 sones. If the subjects are asked to divide the same range of intensity into three equal increments of loudness, they choose successive equal increases of 5 sones at each step, creating an equal-increment loudness scale of approximately 40, 65, 74, and 80 dB SPL. See the discussion in Stevens and Davis (1983) on different attitudes in judging loudness scales.

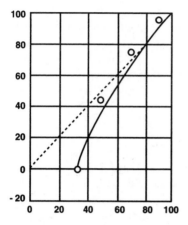 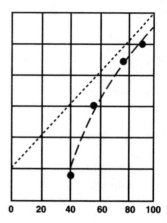

Figure 6–4. Relation between normal loudness function (dashed lines), loudness function for complete recruitment (solid line, left), and loudness function for incomplete recruitment (heavy dashed line, right). Vertical axes represent loudness, horizontal axes intensity. A straight line was chosen to represent the normal loudness function to facilitate comparison with the abnormal loudness functions. (From "The Dependence of Hearing Impairment on Sound Intensity," by J. C. Steinberg and M. B. Gardner, 1937, p. 13. *Journal of the Acoustical Society of America, 9*. Reprinted with permission.)

recruitment. Each loudness function starts at the threshold of hearing; the abnormal functions start at a higher SPL, reflecting an elevated threshold of hearing, and they have an initial slope greater than 45°, indicating that a given change of intensity produces a greater than normal change in loudness. When the recruitment is complete, the impaired- and normal-hearing curves merge at some high level, meaning that the impaired listener hears intense sounds at the same loudness as normal listeners hear them. (Steinberg and Gardner show complete recruitment at 80 dB above threshold, but complete recruitment may occur at other SPL values.) When the recruitment is incomplete, the slope of the loudness function levels off toward the normal reference without reaching it; the loudness response of the impaired-hearing subject improves toward normal as the intensity increases, but never catches up with normal response.

Another way to plot the effects of recruitment is illustrated in Figure 6–5, from an article by Dix, Hallpike, and Hood (1948). These experimenters also used subjects with one normal and one impaired ear. The numbers on the left vertical scales of each diagram of Figure 6–5 are the SPLs of sounds presented to the normal ear, and the numbers on the right vertical scales are the SPLs of sounds presented to the impaired ear. The lines between left and right scales connect the

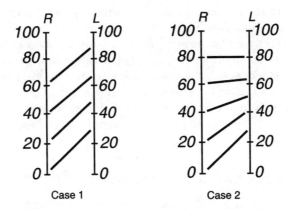

Case 1   Case 2

Figure 6–5. Relation between the SPLs required to produce the same loudness in a normal right ear and an impaired left ear at different stimulus levels to the normal ear. Case 1: conductive impairment. Case 2: cochlear impairment. (From "Observations Upon the Loudness Recruitment Phenomenon, with Especial Reference to the Differential Diagnosis of Disorders of the Internal Ear and VIII Nerve," by M. R. Dix, C. S. Hallpike, and J. D. Hood, 1948, p. 517. *Proceedings of the Royal Society of Medicine.* Reprinted with permission.)

sound-intensity values that produce the same loudness in the impaired ear as in the normal ear, at different stimulus intensities to the normal ear. In Case 1, for a subject with conductive hearing loss and no recruitment, there is a 30-dB difference in threshold SPLs between ears, and at all higher levels the intensity difference between tones required to produce the same loudness in each ear remains at 30 dB. In Case 2, for a subject with a cochlear hearing loss and recruitment, there is also a 30-dB difference in threshold SPLs between ears. As the level is increased, however, there is a successive reduction of the relative intensity of sound that needs to be delivered to the impaired left ear to produce the same loudness as in the normal right ear. At 80 dB above normal threshold, the sound intensity required in the impaired ear to produce the same loudness as in the normal ear is no different than the intensity required in the normal ear, indicating complete recruitment. For this subject with an impaired left ear, a tone 80 dB above threshold produces the same loudness in each ear.

A common misconception about recruitment is that it lowers the tolerance level for intense sound. For example, the fitting instructions of one hearing-aid manufacturer advises using less gain "in cases of severe intolerance for loud sounds (recruitment)." This misconception probably arose from the complaints of patients with recruitment who were given too much linear amplification (amplification in which the gain does not vary with level). A patient with recruitment is likely to hear high-intensity sounds at normal or near-normal loudness unaided, and when the gain of a linear amplifier is set to bring the weak sounds of speech to a comfortable level for the patient, that amount of gain will make high-intensity sounds uncomfortably loud and sometimes unbearable.

The Difference Limen for Intensity

The *just noticeable difference* (jnd) for intensity, also called a *difference limen* for intensity, is the smallest change in sound intensity that can be detected under particular conditions. Figure 6–6, from Riesz (1928), shows that the minimum perceptible intensity difference for normal listeners varies significantly with both frequency and level. The numbers on each curve represent *sensation levels* (the number of dB above threshold); the jnd varies from more than 5 dB just above threshold at 125 Hz, to 0.2 dB at a sensation level of 80 dB over most of the frequency range. Assuming that these data also represent the jnds of hearing-impaired persons, the implication is that the audiologist can

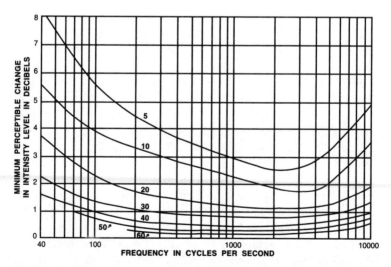

Figure 6–6. Just noticeable difference (jnd) or difference limen for intensity at different frequencies and intensity levels. (From "Differential Intensity Sensitivity of the Ear for Pure Tones," by R. R. Reisz, 1928. *Physical Review 31.*)

expect patients to detect smaller changes of intensity at high sound levels than at levels near threshold. The reduced jnd at high sound levels is consistent with the loudness function of Figure 6–3, which shows that the incremental change of loudness for a given change of intensity is greater at high levels.

It was once thought that persons with recruitment would have smaller jnds for sound intensity.[4] This seems logical, but it has been demonstrated that the intensity jnds of persons with impaired hearing are typically no different from those of normals. Because persons with recruitment have a smaller dynamic range of residual hearing (usually defined as the amplitude range between threshold and discomfort or between threshold and speech levels), they must have a smaller number of jnds within that dynamic range. But misconceptions tend to be long-lived, and the idea that recruitment reduces the jnd, or is even defined by a reduced jnd, persists.[5] In any case, no relationship has been reported between the size of the jnd and speech understanding.

The Physiological Basis for Recruitment

When the recruitment phenomenon was discovered, its physiological basis was not understood. Today we know that it is caused by degeneration of the outer hair cells (Ruggero, 1992). These hair cells, when healthy, process the signal before it gets to the inner hair cells, providing more amplification for weak sounds than for intense sounds. Recruitment may be thought of as a negative effect, an absence of this outer-hair-cell effect. When weak sounds fail to receive the normal extra amplification by outer hair cells in the cochlea, the contrast in loudness between weak and intense sound is exaggerated compared to the normal case.

Recruitment is not characterized by a reduced jnd or by a reduced tolerance for intense sound, but by the recovery or partial recovery of normal loudness response (the loudness induced by a given sound intensity) as sound intensity is increased. The patient has a significant hearing loss for weak sounds but hears intense sounds at normal or

[4]It was at first thought that recruitment would reduce the height of Békésy threshold tracings, which record the interval between the level at which a tone is first heard in a presentation of rising amplitude, and the level at which the tone disappears in a presentation of falling amplitude. But it has turned out that recruitment does not reduce the height of Békésy tracings.

[5]A 1996 article (which shall remain nameless) states: "... individuals having cochlear pathology involving the hair cells are capable of differentiating 1 dB increments. This constitutes 'abnormal growth in the perception of loudness' and defines recruitment." It does neither.

near-normal loudness. Recruitment may also be described as an accelerated loss of loudness as the sound intensity is decreased. Recruitment is to be expected in persons with cochlear impairment involving the outer hair cells, which makes it a typical feature of nonconductive hearing impairment. Recruitment has important implications for hearing-aid amplification (see Chapter 9).

Loudness Relative to Frequency

Figure 6–7 is the well known family of *equal-loudness contours* measured by Fletcher and Munson (1933). Each curve, starting from the reference of a given SPL at 1 kHz, plots the sound intensity that will produce the same loudness at every point of the audible frequency spectrum for an average normal listener. For all reference levels, hearing sensitivity is greatest in the 3 kHz to 4 kHz region (a given loudness requires the least sound intensity), while hearing sensitivity is progressively reduced at low frequencies (a given loudness requires increasing sound intensity as the frequency is lowered). If it takes 70-dB SPL to produce a particular loudness sensation at 1 kHz, it takes about 3 dB less to produce the same loudness at 4 kHz and 10 dB more for the same loudness at 70 Hz. Further, the shape of the contour changes with the 1-kHz reference level, so that relative hearing sensitivity at lower frequencies is reduced as the level of sound is reduced. When we listen to reproduced music at low levels the bass seems to disappear.

Each curve in Figure 6–7 is labelled with a number, which is the *phon* level for all points on that curve.[6] The phon level of a 1-kHz tone is the same as the SPL (in dB re 0.0002 μbar) of the tone; the phon level of a tone at any other frequency is numerically equal to the SPL of a 1-kHz tone that for normal-hearing listeners matches the former in loudness. For example, in the 50-phon equal-loudness contour of Figure 6–7, the SPL at 1 kHz is 50 dB, while the SPL at 200 Hz is 60 dB. A tone of 60-dB SPL at 200 Hz has the same loudness as a tone of 50-dB SPL at 1 kHz, which makes the 200-Hz, 60-dB SPL tone a 50-phon tone. If loudness response did not vary over the frequency spectrum, there would be no need for a phon unit separate from the SPL unit.

[6]The phon level is the *parameter*, or independent variable, of this family of curves; it is the variable whose values represented in the graph are chosen beforehand. The common use of "parameter" to mean any defining characteristic is a careless and improper expropriation of a mathematical term that has a precise meaning.

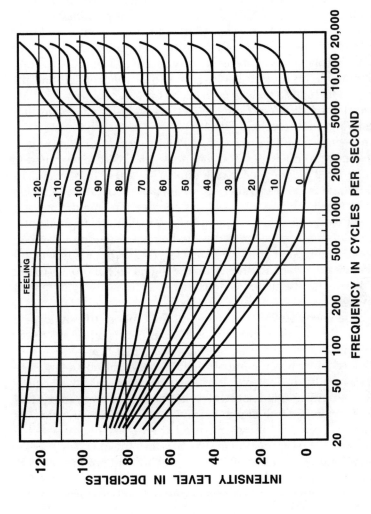

Figure 6–7. Fletcher-Munson equal-loudness contours. (From "Loudness, Its Definition, Measurement and Calculation," by H. Fletcher and W. A. Munson, 1933, p. 91. *Journal of the Acoustical Society of America, 5.* Reprinted with permission.)

The bottom equal-loudness contour, at 0-phon level, represents normal thresholds of hearing in SPLs under particular measurement conditions, while the contours at other levels predict the relative loudness with which normal listeners hear the different sounds of speech and the environment.

Other measurements of equal-loudness contours have been made since the Fletcher-Munson study of 1933, and an international standard for these contours, ISO/R 226 (1961), has been published. The ISO curves represent MAF (see Chapter 2), binaural values, as do the Fletcher-Munson curves, although the latter were not made in the free field but by earphones with a free-field calibration. The ISO measurements were made on subjects between 18 and 25 years of age, and the ISO Standard includes a table of corrections for older subjects. The ISO values are slightly different from the Fletcher-Munson values, including higher values for threshold SPLs.

Sound-level meters measure the SPLs of sounds that may have many frequency components, and the meter readings are weighted to compensate for the dependence of loudness on signal frequency. The American Standard *A* weighting approximates the relative loudness response of the 40-phon equal loudness contour: The main effect is a reduction of readings at low frequencies. A *B* weighting approximates the relative loudness response of the 70-phon equal-loudness contour, with a smaller reduction at low frequencies. A *C* reading is unweighted by the frequency components of the signal except for a rolloff above 5 kHz. The frequency characteristics of these weightings are shown in Figure 6–8.

The difference between the shapes of the 0-phon (threshold) and 70-phon equal-loudness contours of Figure 6–6 is not very great above 700 Hz, but these contours represent normal hearing. For persons with a cochlear hearing impairment there is typically a large difference between the shapes of their threshold curves and their equal-loudness contours at aided speech levels, because of recruitment that varies with frequency (see Figure 9–1 in Chapter 9). Hearing aids are not usually expected to bring impaired thresholds to normal, but more than one fitting system (e.g., ELCVIL and FIG6) is designed to bring equal-loudness contours at the patient's aided speech levels to normal.

A hearing impairment is commonly defined in terms of the patient's threshold SPLs or HLs over the frequency spectrum. But the patient's equal-loudness contours at speech levels bear more directly on his or her ability to hear elements of speech at different levels and frequencies.

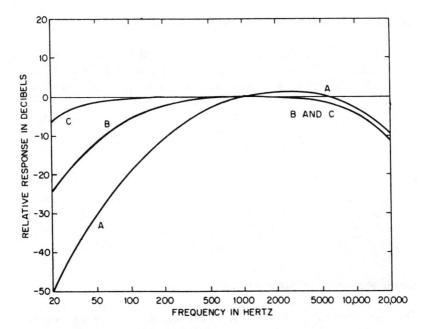

Figure 6–8. Frequency characteristics of *A*, *B*, and *C* weighting of sound level meters. (From "Acoustical Measurement Instruments," by D. L. Johnson, A. M. Marsh, and C. M. Harris, 1998, p. 5.13. In C. M. Harris [Ed.] *Handbook of Acoustical Measurements and Noise.* New York: Acoustical Society of America. Reprinted with permission.)

Loudness Relative to Duration

I once checked a hearing aid driven into its limiting mode of operation by the clicking sound of plastic poker chips hitting one another. The chip sound wasn't very loud because of its short duration—a few milliseconds—but measurement of this sound revealed SPLs above 100 dB, well above the limiting threshold of the hearing aid.

One reason the influence of duration on loudness is of interest to the audiologist is that short, interrupted signals are sometimes used in audiometric testing. All studies of the relation between loudness and duration have not reported the same results, but it is generally accepted that if the duration of test signals is somewhere between 250 and 500 ms, a further increase of signal duration will not significantly increase the signal's loudness.

Loudness Relative to Signal Bandwidth

The *bandwidth* of a signal refers to the range of frequencies occupied by its different elements. The loudness of a signal held at a given overall SPL does not increase when its bandwidth is increased from that of a single-frequency tone to what is called the *critical bandwidth* or *critical band* of frequencies for that frequency region. An increase of bandwidth beyond the critical band, still keeping the total SPL the same, does increase the loudness; the signal then occupies more than one critical band. For normal-hearing persons, the width of the critical band above 500 Hz is roughly one third of an octave, while below 500 Hz the width of the critical band in Hz stays constant at about 100 Hz.

The critical band is also defined as the bandwidth of masker frequencies, sometimes within a broadband masker, that is primarily responsible for masking a tone of a particular frequency.

Loudness and Hearing Impairment

The element of loudness is of prime importance to a hearing-impaired person. The sounds of speech and of the outside world are of course reduced in loudness by the impairment, but this difficulty can usually be corrected by simple amplification. It is the *selective loss* of loudness relative to the amplitudes and the frequencies of different elements of speech—a loss that continues into inaudibility—that is largely responsible for the well known complaint: "I can hear but I can't understand." The selective loss of loudness associated with a combination of recruitment and accentuated high-frequency loss degrades speech intelligibility by making low-amplitude, high-frequency consonants weak or inaudible, but has a much smaller effect on the overall loudness of speech. High-frequency consonants contribute more to the intelligibility of speech (see Figure 7–2) than they do to its total energy (see Figure 7–4).

HEARING PATHOLOGIES OTHER THAN THOSE RELATED TO LOUDNESS

Hearing-impaired persons, particularly those with profound deafness, may have hearing abnormalities that are not a function of their selective loudness response. They may, for example, have a reduced sensitivity to frequency differences, and/or a diminished ability to distinguish temporal (time) gaps. The perception of differences in frequency between successive signals is called *frequency discrimination*, and the perception of differences in frequency between simultaneous signals is called *frequency selectivity*. A loss of frequency discrimination affects the ability to use or interpret normal pitch intonations in speech, in speaking, and in listening, since the intonations can't be heard. A loss of frequency selectivity affects the accurate hearing of formants and formant transitions in speech (see Chapter 7).

Although hearing abnormalities associated with the identification of time and frequency elements in speech may be expected to affect speech recognition, their relation to such recognition has not yet been fully analyzed.

BINAURAL HEARING

Binaural hearing has an effect on both loudness and masking.

The greatest advantage to binaural hearing is the phenomenon called *binaural release from masking*, which is dependent on the differences between sound heard by the left and right ears. It is expressed in decibels as the binaural improvement (decrease) over the monaural masked threshold. It is also called the *masking level difference (MLD)*. For those who like technical jargon, the former term has the disadvantage of being self-explanatory.

Sound reaching the listener from a particular direction will be received differently by each ear. Unless the source of sound is directly in front of, behind, above, or below the listener, the source will be closer to one ear than the other, and there will be differences in the time of arrival and in the intensity of sound at each ear. In addition, except in the special circumstance in which the time delay to the more distant ear is an exact multiple of the period, the sound will arrive at the distant ear at a different point of the individual cycle, and there will be a phase difference between sound at the two ears. Finally, when the sound is not coming from directly ahead, behind, above, or below, the high-frequency emphasis of head diffraction (see curve 1 of Figure 5–1) and the high-frequency attenuation of head shadow will be different for each ear. All of these effects are increased by involuntary head movements.

Although monaural listening provides some sense of direction, the most important factor that allows a listener to identify the direction from which sound is coming is the difference between sounds received at the two ears. These directional cues apply not only to sound radiated directly from a source, but to all of the reflections of that sound in a normally reverberant room. It has been established experimentally that binaural listening has a significant advantage for understanding speech in noise (Hawkins & Yaculo, 1984). At least part of this advantage derives from the increased ability to localize both direct and reflected sound. The audio field can be sensed from the direction from which each ray of direct or reflected sound reaches the ears, and this sense increases the contrast between the target signal and the rest of the field. Localization, however, may or may not be the entire explanation for the binaural release from masking.

A second advantage to listening with two ears rather than one is that sound of a given intensity is louder when heard by both ears, a phenomenon called *binaural loudness summation*. Two-eared listening at threshold has a 2 to 3 dB advantage in loudness for normal-hearing listeners (thresholds are 2 to 3 dB better than for one ear), an advantage that does not vary significantly over the audiometer frequen-cy range. At speech levels there is a 6- to 8-dB binaural increase in loudness for normal listeners. Binaural loudness summation occurs whether the two ears are listening in the natural binaur-al (*dichotic*) mode, or in the *diotic* mode, in which the sound present-ed to each ear is identical (e.g., from earphones connected in parallel).

The increase in loudness created by binaural loudness summation has a particular advantage for hearing-impaired persons, in that a given loudness is produced at a lower sound intensity. This reduces the power requirements for hearing aids, and it also reduces the burden on the ear mechanism, a mechanism that creates distortion at high sound intensities whatever the perceived loudness. Pickett (1973) pointed out that the intelligibility scores of normal-hearing listeners are reduced when speech is presented to them at the high sound levels required by hearing-impaired persons, and suggested that these high sound levels themselves contribute to a loss of intelligibility in hearing-impaired subjects. Because the ear is mechanically nonlinear, it is a reasonable hypothesis that the high sound intensities produced by hearing-aid amplification contribute to the loss of speech intelligibility, and that binaural loudness summation, in reducing the sound intensity required for a given loudness, benefits speech intelligibility. In a binaural fitting, the gain required for each ear is typically reduced about 4 dB from the gain required in a monaural fitting. (Clinical experience has shown that the binaural advantage in loudness at speech levels for hearing-impaired listeners with a cochlear impairment is less than that for normal-hearing listeners.)

A binaural fitting of hearing aids has the additional advantage of serving as a 4-dB buffer against acoustic feedback: The subject's preferred loudness can be achieved with 4 dB less acoustical output from the hearing aid.

A few patients have trouble integrating signals from their left and right ears and do not do well with a binaural fitting. But for the overwhelming majority of patients with hearing impairment in both ears, binaural fitting, outside of questions of cost, has a very significant advantage.

References

Allen, J. B. (1997). A short history of telephone physics. Audio Engineering Society 103rd Convention preprint, pp. 9–15.

American National Institute Standard ANSI S3.20-1973. (1973). *Psychoacoustical terminology* (p. 26). New York: Acoustical Society of America.

Dix, M. R., Hallpike, C. S., & Hood, J. D. (1948). Observations upon the loudness recruitment phenomenon, with especial reference to the differential diagnosis of disorders of the internal ear and VIII nerve. *Proceedings of the Royal Society of Medicine*, 516–526.

Fletcher, H. (1938). Loudness, masking and their relation to the hearing process, and the problem of noise measurement. *Journal of the Acoustical Society of America, 9*, 275–293.

Fletcher, H. (1953). *Speech and hearing in communication* (p. 192). New York: D. Van Nostrand Co.

Fletcher, H., & Munson, W. (1933). Loudness, its definition, measurement, and calculation. *Journal of the Acoustical Society of America, 5*, 82–108.

Fletcher, H., & Munson, W. (1937). Relation between loudness and masking. *Journal of the Acoustical Society of America, 9*, 1–10.

Hawkins, D., & Yacullo, W. S. (!984). Signal-to-noise advantage of binaural hearing aids and directional microphones under different levels of reverberation. *Journal of Speech and Hearing Disorders, 49*, 278–286.

ISO Recommendation R 226. (1961). *Normal equal-loudness contours for pure tones and normal thresholds of hearing under free field listening conditions.* New York: International Organization for Standardization.

Johnson, D. L., Marsh, A. M., & Harris, C. M. (1998). Acoustical measurement instruments. In C. M. Harris (Ed.), *Handbook of acoustical measurements and noise control* (p. 5.13). New York: Acoustical Society of America.

Pickett, J. M. (1973). On discrimination of formant transitions by persons with severe sensorineural hearing loss. In G. Fant & M. A. A. Tatum (Eds.), *Proceedings of a symposium on auditory analysis and perception of speech, Leningrad 1973* (pp. 275–292). London: Academic Press.

Riesz, R. R. (1928). Differential intensity sensitivity of the ear for pure tones. *Physical Review 31*, 867–875.

Ruggero, M. A. (1992). Responses to sound of the basilar membrane of the mammalian cochlea. *Current Opinion in Neurobiology, 2*, 449–456.

Steinberg, J. C., & Gardner, M. B. (1937). The dependence of hearing impairment on sound intensity. *Journal of the Acoustical Society of America 9*, 11–23.

Stevens, S. S. (1955). The measurement of loudness. *Journal of the Acoustical Society of America 27*, 815–829.

Stevens, S. S., & Davis, H. (1983). *Hearing: Its psychology and physiology* (pp. 122–123, 214). New York: American Institute of Physics. [Original publication 1938].

Wever, E. G. (1970). *Theory of hearing* (p. 301). New York: Dover Publications. [Original publication 1949].

Recommended Reading

Fletcher, H. (1953). *Speech and hearing in communication.* New York: D. Van Nostrand Co.

Moore, B. C. J. (1997). *An introduction to the psychology of hearing.* New York: Academic Press.

Stevens, S. S., & Davis, H. (1938, 1983). *Hearing: Its psychology and physiology.* New York: American Institute of Physics.

CHAPTER 7

Music and Speech

MUSICAL INSTRUMENTS

The human voice mechanism and most musical instruments have a similar basic design. In each, a primary vibrating source starts the process of tone generation, and the sound from this primary source is then sent through and changed by a system of resonators and acoustic coupling devices.

The typical primary vibration produces a triangular, "saw-toothed" waveform (a series of these waveforms looks like the edge of a saw) that by itself would sound like a buzzer. It contains energy over a broad range of frequencies and includes an extended series of harmonics. The saw-toothed stimulus is produced in the viol family by the alternate drag and release of a stretched string by a bow coated with rosin, in wind instruments by the periodic interruption of a stream of air, and in brass instruments by the vibration and throttling action of human lips against a mouthpiece. These unmusical stimuli provide the initial oscillatory energy for the fundamental tones and a series of harmonic overtones. The broad range and dense distribution of frequencies in the primary sound is needed because the resonators of musical instruments or of the human voice mechanism are passive devices, and perform their functions only when they receive energy at their own resonance frequencies.

In the case of some percussive instruments, the primary source makes up the major part of the system and the overtones are not harmonic, but usually the source is coupled to and partly controlled by acoustical and/or mechanical resonators that selectively emphasize some overtones and give the sound its characteristic tone color. The sound may also retain a little of the noise component of the primary source—the resinous scrape of the bow or the twang of a plucked string—which gives the listener a sense of how the sound was produced, the way visible brush strokes in a painting give the viewer a sense of how the paint was applied.

The fundamental frequency of the primary waveform is the fundamental frequency of the final tone and therefore defines its pitch. In reedless wind instruments like the flute or flue organ pipe, or in an empty bottle, the fundamental frequency of the primary stimulus is determined almost entirely by the resonators to which it is coupled. The primary vibration of these instruments is produced by directing a steady stream of air against a hard edge; the air flips back and forth across the edge, creating an *edge tone* whose frequency is subject to control by the resonators.

The primary stimulus of bowed strings is also controlled by the resonance of the stretched string. The moving bow drags the string with it until the elastic restoring force of the string overcomes the friction between the bow and the string; the string then springs back until the bow catches it again. The frequency of this drag-and-release operation is controlled by the resonance frequency of the string.

The acoustical resonators of the human voice mechanism, in contrast, control the overtones but have little or no effect on the fundamental frequency of the primary vibration and of the voice.

The majority of musical instruments have a sounding board or horn, which increases their efficiency in radiating sound into the air and also contributes to their tone quality.

THE HUMAN VOICE MECHANISM

Like musical tones, speech is made up of fundamentals and overtones, but it has special characteristics that make it recognizable as language.

The waveform of the primary sound that starts the process of tone generation in the voice mechanism is, as in most musical instruments, usually saw-toothed. For voiced sounds like vowels, the vocal folds or "true" vocal cords (contained in the larynx), driven by a steady flow of air from the lungs, throttle the flow at each cycle to release puffs of air. For intense sounds the cords close completely; for soft sounds they close incompletely. The speaker or singer controls the fundamental frequency of these puffs of air by varying the tension on the vocal cords. The resonating vocal cavities—the pharynx (throat cavity), mouth, and nasal cavity—pick off and reinforce various overtones, giving the sound its tonal structure.

The initial saw-toothed waveform is made up of a fundamental and series of harmonic overtones, which means that the frequency interval between each overtone is the fundamental frequency. But the vocal-tract cavities have their own resonance frequencies (both air-column and Helmholtz), and the cavities provide a rather broad emphasis for those harmonics of the speech signal that lie in the frequency regions of cavity resonances. The cavities are changed by the position of the mouth, tongue, and lips to form vocal-tract resonances unique to each vowel sound; the resulting sounds are defined by their *place of articulation* (i.e., where the resonances are created). Sounds that are formed in different ways, such as stops and fricatives, are distinguished by their *manner* of production.

Vocal-tract resonances are not sharp because damping is provided by the *glottis* (the slit between the vocal folds), viscous losses at the vocal-tract surfaces (friction between air molecules), vibration of the surface tissues, and finally, by the loss of energy when the sound leaves the mouth (see Flanagan, 1972).

SPEECH RECOGNITION

When the saw-toothed output of the vocal cords is modified by the vocal-tract resonators, the effect on the harmonic series of the sound may be represented by the line spectrum of Figure 7–1. As in the violin line spectrum of Figure 1–3, the height of each bar represents the relative amplitude of each harmonic, and the bars are separated by the frequency of the fundamental. The groupings of higher amplitude bars represent the emphasis of those harmonics that occur in the frequency regions of vocal-tract resonances. These emphasized harmonic groupings are called *formants*; the center frequency of the formant region is the *formant frequency*. The lowest frequency resonance of the vocal tract produces the first formant, after which there may be two or three formants successively higher in frequency that are significant to speech recognition. Formants are produced simultaneously with the fundamental, in contrast to the separation in time between vowels and consonants, and unlike the harmonics themselves, formants are rarely spaced evenly in frequency.

The identity of a simple vowel in isolation is strongly dependent on the frequency, amplitude, and bandwidth of its formants; vowels can be synthesized by manipulating these formant elements alone. But

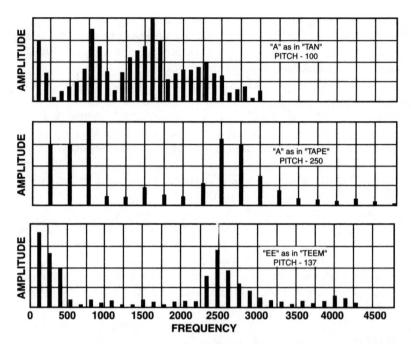

Figure 7–1. Line spectra of different vowel sounds. The height of each bar represents the relative amplitude of each harmonic, and the bars are separated by the frequency of the fundamental, which is the pitch. Note the groupings of higher-amplitude harmonics in the formant frequency regions. (From *Speech and Hearing in Communication,* by H. Fletcher, 1953, p. 52. New York: D. Van Nostrand Co. Reprinted with permission).

vowels have additional acoustical characteristics that are important in the context of speech: shifts in formant-frequency patterns called *formant transitions,* which provide information about adjacent consonants; onset time (i.e., whether the vowel is started abruptly or slowly); and duration.

For unvoiced consonants like /s/ or /f/ (or a whisper), the vocal cords are not involved; for these consonants a steady stream of air is broken up when it is forced through narrow passages formed by the tongue, teeth, and lips. Artificial speech mechanisms produce unvoiced sounds by injecting noise rather than periodic tones. A voiced undertone may be added to an unvoiced consonant to convert /s/ to /z/, /sh/ (ʃ) to /zh/ (ʒ), /f/ to /v/, etc. All of these sounds are called voiced or unvoiced *fricatives.* A *stop* is created by a momentary blockage at some point of the vocal tract; it may be voiced, like /b/ or /d/, or unvoiced, like /p/ or /t/. A fricative combined with a stop, (/sh/ (ʃ) changed to /ch/ (ʧ) is called an *affricative.*

An important part of the acoustic speech signal that makes it recognizable as language is the wave envelope; the time pattern in which the acoustic elements start, change intensity, and stop. In the sound /st/, for example, the steady fricative sound of /s/ is followed by a silent interval, then by the sharp-attack stop /t/; recognition of this time pattern of amplitude changes is necessary in identifying the speech sound.

A *phoneme* is the smallest distinctive, meaningful unit in the sounds of speech: The word /stop/, for example, is made up of four phonemes. Written words and sentences are created by putting a series of phonemic symbols together, usually without further embellishment other than punctuation, but speech is more than a string of phonemes. In addition to stress, duration, pitch intonation (the pattern of pitch changes), and pace—features called *prosodic* or *suprasegmental*—many phonemes carry information about previous or succeeding speech elements, and this information reduces the rate at which discrete sounds must be perceived in order to understand speech (see Liberman, Cooper, Shankweiler, & Studdert-Kennedy, 1967). As noted above, formant transitions contain cues to adjacent consonants, and the duration of a vowel sound is affected by its consonant environment; for example, vowels before stops are longer if the stop is voiced, so that the vowel in /cob/ has a longer duration than in /cop/. Phonemes may be varied by individual and regional pronounciation and still be recognized within their acoustic contexts. These variations are called *allophones*.

Noise and especially reverberation obscure the fine detail of fast changes in the wave envelope, and thus obscure the contribution of these speech elements to intelligibility. A reduced ability in profoundly deaf persons to detect such fast changes would have a similar effect.

The Articulation Index

Speech researchers at Bell Laboratories, notably Fletcher in the 1920s and 1930s and French and Steinberg in their 1947 paper, divided speech into a series of frequency bands, assigning a different importance to the contribution of each band to intelligibility. The application of this analysis to speech transmission provided an index of its intelligibility called the *articulation index* (AI). The AI made it possible to calculate the relative effect of missing or masked frequency bands in different parts of the spectrum of imperfect transmissions or, in the case of listeners with impaired hearing, imperfect perception.

Mueller and Killion (1990) made it easier to use the articulation index to evaluate intelligibility, by applying a graphic system they called "count the dots." The speech cues in different frequency bands

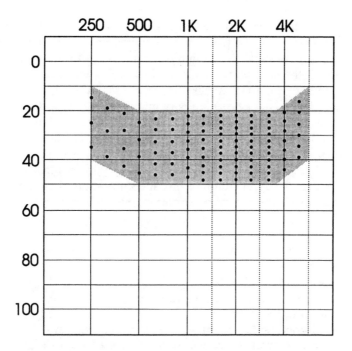

Figure 7–2. "Count-the-dots" system for calculating the Articulation Index. The simplified frequency/amplitude band of speech is plotted in HLs; the number of dots in each column reflects the importance of signals in that frequency region to speech intelligibility. (From "An Easy Method for Calculating the Articulation Index," by G. Mueller and M. C. Killion, 1990, p. 2. *The Hearing Journal, 43.* Reprinted with permission.)

of speech are represented by vertical columns of dots; the number of dots in each band represents the relative importance of that band to speech intelligibility. Figure 7–2, from Mueller and Killion (1990), shows these columns of dots in a simplified frequency/amplitude band plotted in HLs, representing speech at conversational level.

In Figure 7–2 the frequency bands from 1 kHz to just above 3 kHz have a total of 61 dots, while there are only 39 dots total in all of the bands above and below these frequencies. This distribution of dots indicates the special importance to speech understanding of the mid-frequency range. Superimposing either an aided or unaided audiogram on this diagram shows how many and which dots lie above the thresholds of hearing of the subject, indicating what parts of the speech are audible to the subject and how important these parts are to intelligibility. (In this application, however, the AI does not take into account the effect of

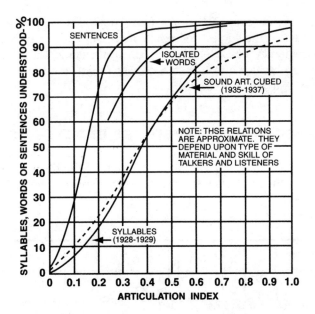

Figure 7-3. Relation between the articulation index and intelligibility on syllable, word, and sentence tests in normal-hearing listeners. High scores are achieved in the sentence tests with a lower articulation index because of additional information from the context of the sentences. (From "Factors Governing the Intelligibility of Speech Sounds," by N. R. French and J. C. Steinberg, 1947, p. 113. *Journal of the Acoustical Society of America, 19.* Re-printed with permission.)

recruitment on the relative loudness of different speech elements.) The articulation index is the number of dots within the audible area divided by the total number of dots (100), and Figure 7–3, from the original paper of French and Steinberg, shows the approximate relation in normal-hearing listeners between the articulation index and intelligibility scores on syllable, word, and sentence tests. French and Steinberg pointed out that sentence scores remain high at low values of the articulation index because the listener can fill in missing sounds by guessing from context, but that the flat portion of the sentence curve is probably accompanied by an appreciable increase of effort.

There are circumstances in addition to the presence of recruitment in which the predictions of the articulation index must be used with caution. A subject with severe mid- and high-frequency loss, for example, may have learned to place more than the usual reliance on low-frequency speech cues. These low-frequency cues become especially important when the subject relies heavily on lipreading, in which case the low-frequency cues, which provide suprasegmental information, have a much greater effect on speech recognition than would be predicted by the articulation index.

THE FREQUENCY/AMPLITUDE BAND OF SPEECH

Figure 7–4, from Villchur (1973), shows part of the dynamic range of hearing over the frequency spectrum, between normal hearing thresh-

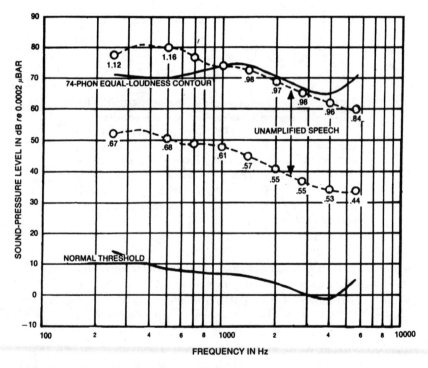

Figure 7–4. Proportionate position, indicated by the numbers on the dashed lines, of the Dunn-White frequency/amplitude band of conversational speech relative to the normal dynamic range of hearing between threshold and the 74-phon ISO equal-loudness contour. The 74-phon contour was chosen for this diagram because it intersects the boundary of high-amplitude levels of speech elements at 1 kHz. (From "Signal Processing to Improve Speech Intelligibility in Perceptive Deafness," by E. Villchur, 1973, p. 1652. *Journal of the Acoustical Society of America, 53.* Reprinted with permission.)

olds in SPLs and the 74-phon normal ISO equal-loudness contour. The 74-phon contour was chosen for this diagram because it intersects the high-amplitude boundary of the Dunn and White (1940)[1] speech band at 1 kHz. Plotted against this frequency/amplitude area of hearing is the frequency/amplitude band of conversational speech, reported separately for male and female voices by Dunn and White but shown here as a composite. The upper speech contour represents speech levels that are exceeded only 1% of the time; the lower speech contour represents levels that are exceeded 80% of the time. The numbers on the dashed lines outlining the speech levels indicate the proportionate position of speech elements at that frequency in the dynamic range of hearing represented.

Even if we extend the bottom of the speech band to cover weaker speech elements, the lowest speech levels lie well above hearing threshold. Discomfort levels are generally reported at about 110 to 115 dB SPL, so that the highest levels of conversational speech lie comfortably below discomfort. These relations will be considered when we discuss the requirements of amplification for hearing-impaired subjects whose residual dynamic ranges of hearing have been reduced by recruitment and accentuated high-frequency loss.

References

Dunn, H. K., & White, S. D. (1940). Statistical measurements on conversational speech. *Journal of the Acoustical Society of America, 11*, 278–288.

Flanagan, J. L. (1972). *Speech analysis synthesis and perception* (pp. 58–69). New York: Springer-Verlag.

Fletcher, H. (1953). *Speech and hearing in communication.* New York: D. Van Nostrand Co.

French, N. R., & Steinberg, J. C. (1947). Factors governing the intelligibility of speech sounds. *Journal of the Acoustical Society of America, 19*, 90–119.

Liberman, A. M., Cooper, F. S., Shankweiler, D. P., & Studdert-Kennedy, M. (1967). Perception of the speech code. *Psychological Review, 74*, 431–461.

Mueller, H. G., & Killion. M. C. (1990). An easy method for calculating the articulation index. *The Hearing Journal 43*, 1–4.

Villchur, E. (1973). Signal processing to improve speech intelligibility in perceptive deafness. *Journal of the Acoustical Society of Amererica, 53*, 1646–1657.

[1]Dunn and White measured conversational speech levels in half-octave bands at the short distance of 30 cm. The limitations of their 1940 equipment prevented them from measuring the lowest levels of speech.

Suggested Reading

Fletcher, H. (1953). *Speech and hearing in communication*. New York: D. Van Nostrand Co.

Kent, R. D., & Read, C. (1992). *The acoustic analysis of speech*. San Diego, CA: Singular Publishing Group.

CHAPTER 8

Amplification

WHAT AN AMPLIFIER DOES

An amplifier is a device that performs an engineering sleight of hand: Its output, the same or almost the same in form as the input, has more energy than was applied at the input. The trick is that energy is borrowed from an outside source and shaped to conform to the input signal. A pipe organ is in a sense an amplifier; the keys control a large flow of air from the bellows, which receive their energy independently. But the first sound amplifier in the modern sense was probably Edison's "aerophone," a pneumatic amplifier illustrated in Figure 8–1. The speaker's voice controlled a sound-actuated valve that in turn controlled the flow of air from an independent source. The air was thus released in vibratory bursts that imitated the speaker's voice, but with more power. Pneumatic amplifiers were used in the early 20th century in phonographs, and were tried as powered megaphones for seaports.

Horns, mechanical levers, and electric transformers all seem to have more output than input, but they are not amplifiers because they do not increase the power of the system. They cannot, because they have no outside source of energy; they can only improve the efficiency with which the input stimulus engages its load.

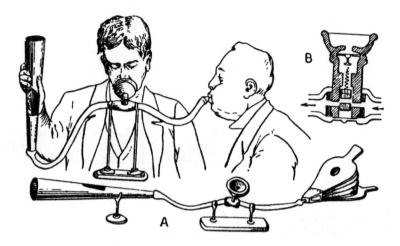

Figure 8–1. Edison's "aerophone," a pneumatic amplifier. A valve was controlled by the speaker's voice; the valve in turn controlled the instantaneous flow of compressed air.

HEARING-AID AMPLIFIERS

In the first hearing-aid amplifiers, used in the 1920s, the power-shaping element was the carbon in the microphone. At moments when the microphone diaphragm exerted pressure on the carbon granules in response to the instantaneous stimulus of a speech waveform, the electrical resistance of the carbon was decreased and more current could flow from the battery to the receiver, as in a telephone; when the diaphragm released its pressure, less current flowed. Carbon amplifiers in hearing aids were followed by miniature-vacuum-tube amplifiers, which were practical because the amplifier and the large battery were worn in a pocket or some other place in the clothing rather than at the ear. The design of the modern hearing aid was made possible first by the transistor and then by the integrated-circuit chip, by improvements in battery technology, and by miniature, high-quality microphones and receivers.

The electronic hearing aid is called on to produce very high sound pressures at the eardrum, sometimes exceeding 125 dB SPL for persons with severe hearing impairment. It is able to do this with a few milliwatts of electrical power driving a tiny receiver because it only needs to service a small volume of air, and because of the technical sophistication of hearing-aid transducers and amplifiers.

CLASSES OF OPERATION

In an electronic amplifier the input stimulus controls current flow from an independent source of power, and the instantaneous value of the current is made to follow the waveform of an alternating signal such as speech. The *class* of operation of a vacuum tube or transistor circuit determines when and how much current is drawn from the power source relative to different parts of the signal cycle and to no-signal intervals. Current that flows during no-signal periods does no useful work and is dissipated in heat.

In class A, as in other classes of operation, the current increases during positive halves of the signal cycle and decreases during negative halves, but in class A the varying flow of current from the power source never stops. The current during no-signal intervals is kept high enough so that when a high-amplitude signal demands large current swings, the instantaneous value of the current can follow the negative half of the signal cycle without being driven to zero and cutoff. The value of the current must also be able to follow the positive half of the cycle without exhausting the capability of the power supply. A higher average value of current is drawn than in any other class of operation; class A is the least efficient class in that it wastes the most current. Class A circuits are rarely used in modern hearing aids because the battery does not last long enough.

Class AB operation (a modified version of class B), which draws very little current when no signal is present, is made possible by the push-pull circuit. The current in each half of a push-pull pair of transistors (or, in previous days, vacuum tubes) is alternately allowed to be driven past cutoff by the signal, so that no current flows for part of the cycle in that half of the circuit; each deficient half cycle is filled in by current from the other member of the push-pull pair. The system is like that of a two-man saw whose operators each have a strong push and a weak pull: The force of push plus pull in each direction is the same. This mode of operation makes possible low distortion and reduced battery drain at the same time.

Class C circuits switch the current off completely during part of the cycle and are very efficient. They are suitable for creating the carrier waves of radio transmissions, but not for audio signals.

In class D circuitry, an invention of the 1940s redesigned by Killion and Carlson to apply to the low-voltage amplifiers of hearing aids (Carlson, 1988; Killion, 1986), the input signal controls the output current indirectly, by controlling a supersonic-frequency, rectangular series of waveforms that act as a carrier for the audio signal. The rectangular waveforms are produced by alternately switching each of a pair of out-of-phase transistors on and off. In the absence of an audio signal, the receiver has no mechanical response to the carrier because of the carrier's supersonic frequency, and because the receiver has a high electrical impedance at the carrier frequency it accepts very little current. But when an audio signal is present, the audio-frequency waveforms control the average value of the supersonic carrier. They do this by varying the relative duration of the positive and negative halves of the carrier's rectangular waveforms—the relative amount of time each of the out-of-phase transistors are on or off—so that for each positive or negative half of the audio cycle the carrier has a net positive or negative average value. This type of control of a carrier for the transmission of signals is called *pulse-width* or *pulse-duration* modulation.

The receiver cannot respond to the steady carrier but it can respond to the audio-frequency variations of the carrier, because during each half of the audio cycle the supersonic impulses are all in the same direction. The receiver responds to the sum of successive net values of the rectangular waveforms and filters out the supersonic component.

Current drain in a class D amplifier is reduced because almost no current is drawn during no-signal periods and because of the way current is controlled to represent the audio signal. When the instantaneous value of the current must be reduced to follow the audio waveform, the class D circuit reduces the average value of its supersonic carrier without wasting power; when current is reduced in class A or class AB operation, power is dissipated in the transistor.

A properly designed Class D circuit allows large swings of the average value of the carrier without reducing the average current below cutoff on negative halves of the audio cycle, or exhausting the current capability of the power supply on positive halves. It therefore handles high-intensity signals well. It combines the low distortion of Class A and Class AB amplifiers with minimum current drain. Killion (in Johnson and Killion, 1994) reported that battery life is extended 30% to 40% compared to a class AB circuit of equal performance.

HARMONIC DISTORTION

The characteristic distortion of electronic amplifiers produces a series of harmonic overtones that are not present in the input signal. The spurious harmonics themselves do not have as great an irritation value as might be supposed; they are, after all, harmonically related in a musical sense to the fundamental, and they may serve to intensify or weaken natural harmonics that already exist. Yet harmonic distortion is raucous and very unpleasant.

This raucous quality derives largely from an effect of harmonic distortion called *intermodulation distortion*, which is created when two or more tones are passed simultaneously through a device with harmonic distortion. If a low-frequency waveform drives an amplifying stage into distortion, the wrong instantaneous amount of current, relative to the dictates of the low-frequency input signal, flows through the tube or transistor. At that moment the amplifier provides either exaggerated or diminished response to *all* stimuli, and any high-frequency signal that is present will be affected. When a complex tone consisting of both low- and high-frequency tones is amplified by such a device, the intermodulation distortion will introduce signals at new frequencies equal to the sums of and differences between the frequencies of the original signals,[1] as shown in Figure 8–2. These frequencies are harmonically unrelated to the original signal frequencies, and the new signals have an abrasive effect, like the adjacent keys of a piano.

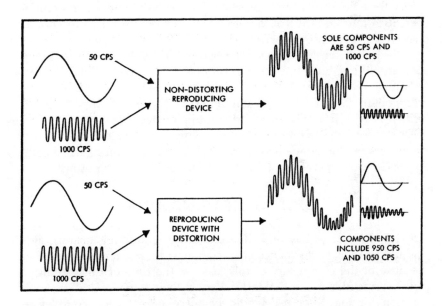

Figure 8-2. Intermodulation distortion created by harmonic distortion of the low-frequency waveform. The wave envelope of the high-frequency signal is amplitude-modulated and contains new signal components. (From *Reproduction of Sound*, by E. Villchur, 1965, p. 16. New York: Dover Publications. Reprinted with permission.)

[1]The amplitude-modulated signal at the lower half of Figure 8–2 can be analyzed into separate frequency components that include 950 Hz and 1050 Hz. The analysis can also be applied in the other direction: If signals at 1000 Hz and 950 Hz (or 1000 Hz and 1050 Hz) are mixed, they will reinforce and cancel each other every 50 Hz, creating the modulation of the 1000 Hz signal shown in Figure 8–2.

DIGITAL AMPLIFIERS

In digital amplifiers, as in class D circuits, the input signal exerts its control over the flow of output current indirectly. The signal is broken up into many segments, and each segment directs the amplifier to reproduce, at the same point of the waveform and the same instant, a segment of the same relative amplitude.

The startling clarity of the photographs sent from Mars was made possible by digital technology. The great distance and interfering electromagnetic fields between Mars and Earth made an ordinary video transmission impractical. With digital transmission, the camera on Mars in effect sent out numbers to represent the color and shade of each dot on a synchronized grid on Earth. Electrical interference might make the receiver on Earth miss a number, which would leave a blank space for a dot, but would not make the receiver get the wrong number. Such interference would not be recorded because it would not be received as an appropriate number.

A digital amplifier does not perform a different task from previous amplifiers, but performs the same task differently. It has a great advantage when the medium of communication itself has a large noise component (a noise component independent of the input signal), which is why it works so well for interplanetary transmission, why CDs do not have the surface noise of vinyl records, and why digital tape does not have tape hiss. It also has a clear advantage when complex electronic operations are to be performed, as in computing.

DIGITAL HEARING AIDS

Digital technology has proved useful in programming hearing aids (adjusting their performance characteristics) from a remote controller because of the complexity of this task. At the time of this writing, a few hearing aids use digital technology in their actual operation. Justification for the latter use would be for operations too complex to accomplish easily in analog circuits, and I am not aware of effective processing in use today that cannot be accomodated by analog technology. (An "analog" circuit is the nondigital kind that has been used all these years. After we are introduced to poetry, we learn that what we have been speaking is called prose.) The potential advantage for digital technology in hearing aids may, of course, increase in the future, when we have learned to improve the performance of hearing aids with more complex signal processing.

Possibly the silliest thing I have seen written about digital hearing aids appeared in the medical newsletter of a prestigious medical journal: "Analog hearing aids amplify all sounds, while the programmable, digital models contain circuitry that helps sort out and suppress background noise."

The only noise-suppression circuitry employed in current digital hearing aids does not "sort out" background noise (the difficulties of such processing are discussed in Chapter 10), but simply reduces low-frequency gain in the presence of all low-frequency, high-amplitude signals, whether speech or noise. This circuit design is based on the rationale that interfering noise commonly occurs at low frequencies, that most of the intelligibility-bearing elements of speech are at high frequencies, and that low-frequency noise is more damaging to speech understanding than is the loss of low-frequency speech cues. Processing of this type, which is used in at least one digital aid, is not tied to digital operation and is also used in some analog hearing aids. The writer of the newsletter quoted above may have been confused by the effectiveness with which digital technology has dealt with noise in a transmission or recording medium when the noise is not part of the input signal. There is no advantage to digital technology in dealing with the problem of noise when the noise is part of the input signal, at least until or unless processing too complex for analog circuitry is designed that can separate wanted from unwanted input to the hearing aid. The digital video transmitter on Mars received an uncontaminated input signal before the signal's noisy journey through space. The external noise that enters the microphone of a hearing aid—other people talking, or environmental noise—is part of the input signal and will be treated in more detail in Chapter 10.

References

Carlson, E. V. (1988). An output amplifier whose time has come. *Hearing Instruments, 39,* 30, 32.

Johnson, W. A., & Killion, M. C. (1994, March). Amplification: Is class D better than class B? *American Journal of Audiology,* pp. 11–13. (A debate).

Killion, M. C. (1986). Class D hearing aid amplifier. U.S. Patent 4,592,087.

Villchur, E. (1965). *Reproduction of sound* (p. 16, 46). New York: Dover Publications.

CHAPTER 9

Signal Processing in Hearing Aids

Up to this point in the book I have presented acoustical information that I do not consider controversial. This chapter includes analyses on which a consensus does not exist.

Conductive hearing loss may be compared to a plug blocking the ear canal. If adequate relief cannot be provided medically and hearing aids are used, simple amplification with no processing other than frequency-response shaping is normally all that is needed.

It used to be commonly accepted that "nerve deafness" could not be helped by hearing aids. The people who gave this advice may have been right for nerve deafness, but what they usually meant by nerve deafness was any nonconductive hearing impairment. The typical nonconductive impairment does not involve the acoustic nerve but the hair cells of the cochlea, and patients with that kind of impairment can be helped by hearing aids.

The great majority of the hearing-impaired population have a cochlear impairment that creates both a frequency-selective loss, usually with greater loss at high frequencies, and an amplitude-selective loss (recruitment) with greater loss for weaker signals. Because of the selective nature of these hearing losses, some elements of speech that contain important cues to intelligibility remain inaudible to the patient after undistorted but unprocessed amplification to the patient's preferred level.

The most fundamental task in improving speech intelligibility for a person with a cochlear impairment (sometimes referred to as sensorineural impairment, although it is sensory, not neural) is to amplify as many elements of speech as possible to a level clearly audible by that person. It is obvious that speech elements that cannot be heard by the subject cannot contribute to speech understanding. It is also important, particularly from the point of view of natural sound quality, that as far as possible each speech element—strong or weak, high frequency or low frequency—be amplified to a relative level in the residual dynamic range of hearing of the subject comparable to the relative level of that element in the normal dynamic range of hearing. Comparable relative intensity levels imply comparable loudness levels.

Three kinds of signal treatment are necessary (although not always sufficient) to achieve these goals: (1) amplification that compensates for the increase of hearing loss for weak signals (compression); (2) amplification that simultaneously compensates for the increase of hearing loss in some frequency regions (frequency-response shaping); and (3) adjustment of this signal processing for each subject so that speech signals are amplified to their proper position in the subject's residual dynamic range of hearing over the useful frequency range.

Research in signal processing for the hearing impaired has often failed to include all three of these elements in combination, and I believe this explains some of the inconsistent results of compression and other signal-processing experiments. Either of the first two elements, with or without the third, is a necessary but insufficient condition for success. To draw an analogy with compensation for defective eyesight, subjects with both myopia and astigmatism need adjustment of the focal lengths of their corrective lenses to compensate for their myopia, plus shaping of the lenses to compensate for their astigmatic distortion. Either procedure by itself will be much less effective than the two combined, and the use of both procedures in combination will not be meaningful unless focal lengths and astigmatic corrections are accurately adjusted to the needs of the individual subject.

The reader is referred to Figure 7–4 of Chapter 7, which plots the relation between the frequency/amplitude band of conversational speech and the dynamic range of normal hearing for speech. This dynamic range is defined as the area between the threshold curve in SPLs and an equal-loudness contour at the subject's preferred level for listening to speech[1] over the range of speech frequencies. In Figure 9–1

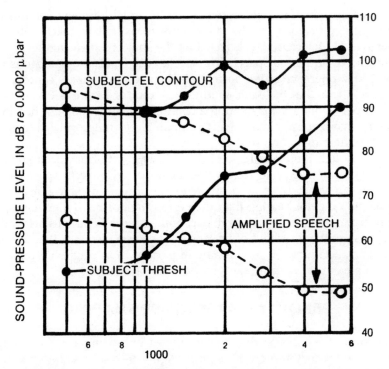

Figure 9–1. The Dunn-White conversational-speech band plotted against the average residual dynamic range of hearing (for aided speech) of six hearing-impaired subjects. The dynamic range is defined as the range between threshold and an equal-loudness contour anchored at 1 kHz to the average preferred amplified-speech level of the subjects. Threshold and equal-loudness measurements were made with an earphone with free-field calibration to match the free-field speech measurements. (From "Simulation of the Effect of Recruitment on Loudness Relationships in Speech," by E. Villchur, 1973, p. 1603. *Journal of the Acoustical Society of America, 56.* Reprinted with permission.)

the same speech band, amplified to the average preferred level of six hearing-impaired subjects from a study by Villchur (1973), is plotted against the average dynamic range of hearing (as defined above, but for amplified speech) of those subjects. The threshold curve is the

[1]The dynamic range of hearing defined here—the area between threshold and an equal-loudness contour at the subject's preferred speech level—is in contrast to the more commonly cited dynamic range of hearing between threshold and discomfort. The former is more suitable for plotting the effects of compression on speech perception, because part of the dynamic range between high-amplitude speech levels and discomfort levels is likely to lie above the level of complete recruitment.

average of their threshold curves, and the equal-loudness contour is the average of equal-loudness contours measured for each subject, using 1-kHz reference levels based on the subject's preferred level for listening to amplified speech. These reference levels are analogous to the 1-kHz reference of the normal 74-phon equal-loudness contour of Figure 7–4, so that the equal-loudness contour of Figure 9–1 serves as the upper boundary for plotting a residual dynamic range of hearing for the average impaired subject comparable to the normal dynamic range of hearing of Figure 7–4.

Although the overall speech level in Figure 9–1 has been amplified to the average preferred level of the impaired subjects, speech levels have a very different position in the impaired-subject residual dynamic range of hearing than they do in the normal dynamic range of hearing of Figure 7–4. A large part of the speech band falls below or too close to the threshold of hearing, and speech elements that the AI diagram of Figure 7–2 predicts are important to intelligibility remain inaudible or too weak after unprocessed amplification.

FREQUENCY-RESPONSE SHAPING

One kind of processing that has been used in hearing aids for a long time is frequency-response shaping. Figure 9–2 shows the effect of high-frequency emphasis on the speech band; the emphasis adjusted as well as it can be to the residual dynamic range of hearing shown in the diagram. Frequency-selective amplification has changed the shape but not the dynamic range of the speech band. It has placed the high-amplitude elements of speech at levels that have approximately the same relation to the subject's equal-loudness contour as the high-amplitude levels of unamplified speech have to the corresponding normal equal-loudness contour, and it is reasonable to expect that these amplified speech elements will have the same loudness and comfort for the impaired subject as the unamplified high-amplitude elements have for a normal listener. But the weaker elements of speech in the high-frequency region remain below threshold, even though 24 dB of extra high-frequency gain has been applied. A comparison of Figure 9–2 with Figure 7–4 also shows that a good part of the speech band, especially in the high-frequency region, has received inadequate amplification in that it lies too close to the threshold of hearing.

The high-frequency emphasis in Figure 9–2 has restored some of the speech elements to audibility and may therefore be expected to improve speech intelligibility, but it has left other speech elements below threshold or too weak. It would take more than 40 dB of extra amplification for the weakest high-frequency speech elements to reach

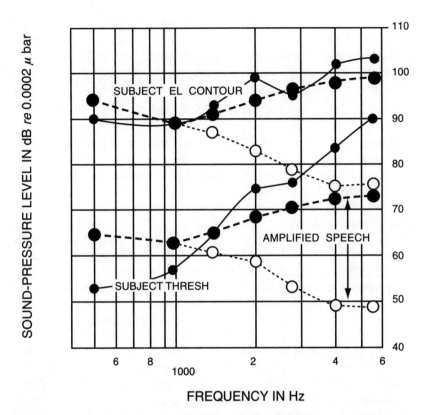

Figure 9–2. The effect of high-frequency emphasis on the speech band. The high-amplitude elements of speech are amplified to a level, relative to the equal-loudness contour, comparable to the level of unaided speech relative to a normal equal-loudness contour (see Figure 7–4), but no compression is used.

relative levels in the residual dynamic range of hearing comparable to the relative levels of those weak elements in the normal dynamic range of hearing. That amount of amplification would become intolerable to the subject when high-amplitude elements of speech or other high-intensity sounds made their appearance.

Skinner (1980) reported experimental results that suggest the same conclusion. She found that high-frequency emphasis improved the speech recognition of her hearing-impaired subjects, but that the higher the presentation level of the speech the less the amount of high-frequency emphasis that was most effective for the subject or that the subject would tolerate.

A large part of the problem could be solved theoretically by manual controls that allow the listener to adjust both gain and high-frequency emphasis with the changing input level of speech to the hearing aid. Adjusting such controls would be a nuisance for slow changes in overall level (different talkers, for example), extremely difficult for sentence-to-sentence changes, and impossible for simultaneous signals or for fast word-to-word or within-word changes.

COMPRESSION

Steinberg and Gardner (1937) concluded their paper on recruitment with this comment: "Owing to the expanding action of this type of loss it would be necessary to introduce a corresponding compression in the amplifier."

Compression, also called *automatic gain control (AGC)*, became for a time a buzz word representing not what Steinberg and Gardner had meant—increased gain at lower sound levels to satisfy the increasing gain demands of recruitment at lower levels—but *limiting*, an electronic ceiling that does not allow the output of a hearing aid to substantially exceed a predetermined level but that has no effect on gain at lower levels. Comparisons between the output versus input characteristics of a compression limiter and of a compressor that covers the dynamic range of speech are shown in Figures 9–3 and 9–4.

For the wide–dynamic-range compressor represented in Figures 9–3 and 9–4, the input level at which compression begins to operate, called the *compression threshold*, is chosen by the compressor designer as the level of the weak elements of speech, in this case about 40 dB SPL. At 40 dB input to this compressor the output is 70 dB, a gain of 30 dB, but as the input is increased above the 40-dB level, the output increases at a slower rate. At 70 dB input to the compressor, the output has only increased to 80 dB SPL. The gain has been reduced from 30 dB to 10 dB. Another way of putting it is that a 30-dB increase of input signal to the compressor produces an increase in output of only 10 dB.

For the compression limiter, on the other hand, the level at which compression begins to operate is chosen as some level above the high-amplitude elements of conversational speech, in Figures 9–3 and 9–4 about 85 dB input SPL. The severe compression in limiting, represented by the reduced slope of the output curve, is virtually a clamp on further output rather than a gradual reduction of output. The limiting provides no extra gain at low input levels that would bring the weak elements of speech to audibility, but does protect the user against discomfort. With very clean (low distortion) limiters, the user may turn up the gain for weaker speech elements and crowd the higher level elements against the limiter ceiling.

The amount of compression is defined by the *compression ratio*, which is the change in dB of input-signal level divided by the result-

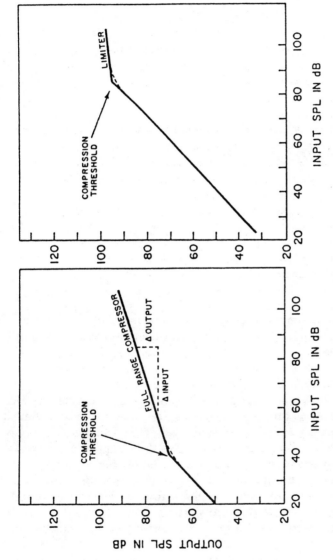

Figure 9–3. Input/output curves showing compression ratios (Δoutput/Δinput) and compression thresholds of wide-dynamic-range compression and of compression limiting. (After "Signal Processing," by E. Villchur, 1978b, p. 225. In M. Ross and T. G. Giolas [Eds.]. *Auditory Management of Hearing Impaired Children.* Baltimore: University Park Press.)

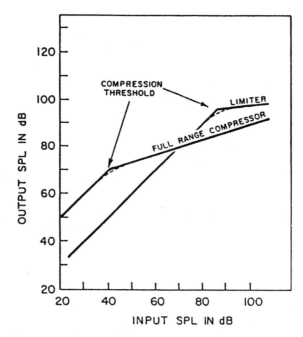

Figure 9–4. The input/output curves of Figure 9–3 plotted on the same graph.

ing change in dB of output-signal level. If the input signal is increased or decreased 10 dB and the resulting increase or decrease in output is only 5 dB, the compression ratio is 2. The compression ratios used in the diagrams of Figures 9-3 and 9-4 are 3 for the wide–dynamic-range compressor and about 8 for the limiter.

Two additional features of compression, which are tied to each other, are the attack time and the release time. *Attack time* is the time it takes a compressor to reduce amplifier gain after a sudden increase of input level; *release time* is the time it takes the compressor to increase amplifier gain after a sudden decrease of input level.[2] Instantaneous attack and release are not used, because instantaneous compression would respond to amplitude changes within the waveforms of individual cycles and create severe distortion. Compressors designed to compensate for recruitment respond to short-term level changes with-

[2]From ANSI Standard S3.22-1996: "The attack time is defined as the time between the abrupt increase from 55 to 90 dB SPL and the point where the level has stabilized to within 3 dB of the steady value for the 90-dB input SPL. The release time is defined as the interval between the abrupt drop from 90 to 55 dB SPL and the point where the signal has stabilized to within 4 dB of the steady-state value for the 55-dB input SPL."

in speech and generally have attack times of a few milliseconds and release times in the range of 40 to 100 ms. Such fast-acting compressors are sometimes called "syllabic" compressors. While they do respond to intensity changes between syllables, they also respond to intensity changes within a syllable; they will change gain three times within a single syllable like "bath." Their action is more appropriately called phonemic compression.

Figure 9–5 shows the effect of compression on the speech band, the compression adjusted to the reduced dynamic range of hearing of the subject. Compression ratios are adjusted separately for low-frequency and high-frequency regions, but no post-compression frequency-response shaping has been added. Figure 9–2 showed that high-frequency emphasis without compression failed to bring many missing elements of speech to audibility, and Figure 9–5 shows that for the same subject, compression without post-compression high-frequency emphasis also fails in this task. In each case, the incomplete processing

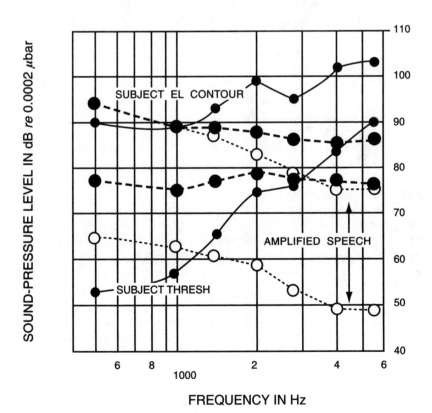

Figure 9–5. The effect of processing the speech band by compression alone, without fixed high-frequency emphasis.

restores only part of the speech band to audibility and to its proper position within the subject's residual dynamic range of hearing. Some of the published experiments that reported little or no benefit to hearing-impaired subjects from compression have used compression processing without post-compression frequency-response shaping.

COMPRESSION COMBINED WITH FREQUENCY-RESPONSE SHAPING

We may now address the problem posed in Figure 9–1 by processing the speech with a combination of wide–dynamic-range compression and post-compression high-frequency emphasis, each adjusted to the residual dynamic range of hearing of the individual impaired subject over the frequency spectrum. This was the system proposed by Villchur (1973),[3] and Figure 9–6 shows the speech band processed in this way, plotted against the average residual dynamic range of hearing of his subjects. Compression has squeezed the speech band—more at high frequencies than at low frequencies because the speech has to fit into a narrower dynamic range of hearing—and high-frequency emphasis has bent the compressed speech band upward, so that most of the speech elements are amplified to a relative level in the dynamic range of hearing of the subject close to their proportionate positions in the normal dynamic range of hearing.

Note that the high-amplitude elements of speech in Figure 9–6 have been amplified to the same level as in the noncompressed frequency-response processing of Figure 9–2. The goal of a compression system is not to reduce the levels of high-amplitude signals, but to amplify high-amplitude signals to their optimum levels for the subject and then to increase the relative gain for low-amplitude signals.

COMPRESSION AND THE GAIN RULE

When hearing-aid performance became flexible enough that the fitter could adjust the overall gain and to some extent the frequency response of the aid, attempts were made to "mirror the audiogram," to provide an amount of gain at each frequency equal to the thresh-

---

[3]The equipment design of the Villchur 1973 experiment was translated to a wearable hearing aid (the Resound) by a team at AT&T Bell Laboratories that included Fred Waldhauer, who was responsible for the basic chip design (Waldhauer & Villchur, 1988), Jont Allen (Allen, 1996), Joseph L. Hall, and Vincent Pluvinage (Pluvinage, 1994).

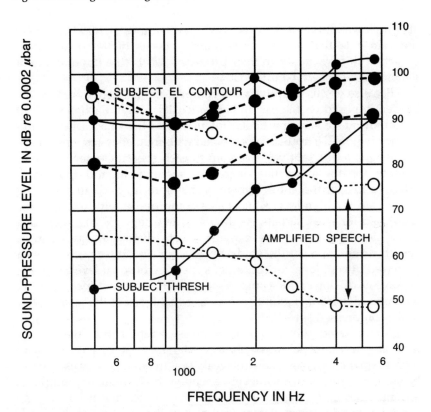

Figure 9–6. The effect of processing the speech band by compression combined with post-compression, high-frequency emphasis. The compression and the high-frequency emphasis are adjusted to fit the speech into the residual dynamic range of hearing of the individual subject, at levels proportionate to the levels of unamplified speech in the normal dynamic range of hearing.

old hearing loss at that frequency. It became apparent that this amount of gain in a noncompression hearing aid would not be tolerated by the patient (except perhaps one with a purely conductive loss); the typical patient has recruitment and requires far less gain at speech levels than at threshold levels. A compromise was worked out defined by a gain rule, a prescription for the amount of desirable gain at each frequency for a linear hearing aid. The gain was calculated as a percentage—commonly 25% to 50%—of the hearing loss in dB at that frequency. The gain rule provided too little gain at low levels for a person with recruitment, and often too much gain at high levels.

Pluvinage (1994) has pointed out that wide–dynamic-range compression follows an adaptive gain rule, high for low-level inputs and low for high-level inputs. For example, in Figure 9–6 the gain rule that lifts the lowest levels of the unamplified speech to their processed levels (the lower curve of the processed speech band) at 1.5 kHz is 59%; the gain rule that amplifies the highest levels of the unamplified speech at this frequency to their processed levels (the upper curve of the processed speech band) is 32%.

Because of this adaptive gain, compression is likely to reduce the burden imposed on the ear by high-intensity sound. Each element of speech or music has a particular intensity and lies in a particular frequency region. Compression combined with frequency-response shaping assigns a different value of gain to each speech element, to compensate for the particular degree of recruitment and frequency-selective loss of the subject; there is therefore no need to allow too much gain for high-level signals as a compromise with the need for more gain for weak signals. As discussed in Chapter 6, high objective sound levels overload the ear and create distortion that reduces speech recognition. In the study by Villchur (1973), subjects chose a preferred overall level for continuous speech whose vu levels were on average 3 dB lower for compressed speech than for linear speech, although higher intelligibility scores were achieved at the lower levels of the compressed speech.

A compressor with a higher compression ratio at high frequencies than at low frequencies assigns a greater increase of gain to weak high-frequency signals than to weak low-frequency signals, as can be seen in Figure 9–5. Such level-dependent high-frequency emphasis is sometimes given the acronym TILL (treble increase at low levels). Most hearing-impaired persons with recruitment require the level-dependent high-frequency emphasis that compression provides, plus the level-independent emphasis of post-compression frequency-response shaping. The latter lifts the high-frequency portion of the compressed speech band to its proper position in the residual dynamic range of hearing in the high-frequency region. The difference between the diagrams of Figures 9–5 and 9–6 is the addition, in Figure 9–6, of level-independent high-frequency emphasis to the level-dependent high-frequency emphasis in Figure 9–5.

The combination of compression and high-frequency emphasis in Figure 9–6 increases the vulnerability of a hearing aid to acoustic feedback. Compression increases the gain for weak high-frequency signals, which can get acoustic feedback started, and the fixed high-frequency emphasis adds to the problem. With this type of processing, greater care is needed in the mechanical fitting.[4]

---

[4]Precautions against acoustic feedback, in addition to care in the physical fit of the earmold or hearing aid, may include the use of foam washers over the canal section of the aid that improve the acoustic seal. These washers are available commercially and can be effective.

MULTICHANNEL COMPRESSION

There are two reasons for using more than one frequency channel of compression. The first is that different frequency regions need different amounts of compression, as discussed above. Recruitment is typically greatest at high frequencies, making the residual dynamic range of hearing at high frequencies smaller than at low frequencies. The speech band therefore needs to be compressed more at high frequencies, which is to say needs a higher compression ratio (Villchur, 1973). Villchur used independent compressors for separate frequency bands in order to allow each band to be adjusted to an appropriate compression ratio. It was this design that produced the processing of Figure 9–6. But there are also compressor designs that can vary the compression ratios for different frequency regions using only one channel of compression. The original was the K-Amp design of Killion (1993), now in common use. It has the advantages of simplicity and lower cost.

The second reason for using more than one frequency channel of compression is that the compressor is sometimes called on to process more than one signal at the same time, each of which lies in a different frequency region and each of which requires different or even opposite treatment. For example, we would want a compressor to reduce gain for high-amplitude, low-frequency noise, while we would want the compressor to increase gain for a low-amplitude, high-frequency consonant present at the same moment. Speech formants are another example of simultaneous signals in different frequency regions that require different amounts of compressor action. A compressor-controlled amplifier can have only one value of gain at any instant (outside of frequency-response variations), and so within a single compressor channel the compressor cannot treat two simultaneous signals differently. It responds only to the highest-amplitude signal present in the channel at that moment.

How significant the multichannel capabilities of a compressor are to impaired-subject intelligibility has not been settled. Many of the intensity contrasts in speech that need to be ameliorated by compression, while they occur in different frequency regions, occur successively rather than simultaneously. I favor separate compression control in different frequency channels.

COMPRESSION AND UNILATERAL RECRUITMENT

The effect of compression may be looked at from another point of view than that in Figure 9–5. Early studies of recruitment used subjects with one normal-hearing ear and one impaired ear, and the

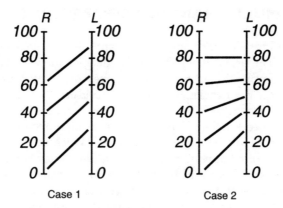

Case 1   Case 2

Figure 9–7. (Repeat of Fig. 6–5). Relation between the SPLs required to produce the same loudness in a normal right ear and an impaired left ear at different stimulus levels to the normal ear. Case 1: conductive impairment. Case 2: cochlear impairment. (From "Observations Upon the Loudness Recruitment Phenomenon, With Especial Reference to the Differential Diagnosis of Disorders of the Internal Ear and VIII Nerve," by M. R. Dix, C. S. Hallpike, and J. D. Hood, 1948, p. 517. *Proceedings of the Royal Society of Medicine.* Reprinted with permission.)

experimenters measured the differences in the intensity of signals required to produce the same loudness in each ear at different stimulus levels, as illustrated in Figure 6–4 of Chapter 6 and shown again in this chapter as Figure 9–7. In case 1 of Figure 9–7—conductive deafness without recruitment in the impaired ear—a constant 30-dB intensity difference between signals to the normal and to the impaired ear is required to produce the same loudness in each ear at all stimulus levels. This calls for linear amplification for the impaired ear: the same amount of gain at all input levels. In Case 2—cochlear deafness with complete recruitment at 80 dB above threshold in the impaired ear—the difference between the intensity of signals that produce the same loudness in normal and impaired ears is progressively reduced as the stimulus to the normal ear is increased, until at 80-dB sensation level the same intensity of sound produces the same loudness in each ear. A different value of gain for the impaired ear is required at each stimulus level, with no gain at 80 dB. Ideally, the gain at each level would make the connecting line at that level horizontal. This variation of gain with input level can only be produced by a compression amplifier or by lightning-quick fingers on the volume control.

The family of connecting lines in Figure 9–7 represents the degree of recruitment at only one frequency. Recruitment typically increases at higher frequencies, so that uniform compression over the frequency range will not keep the lines horizontal at all frequencies. Frequency-dependent compression ratios are required, and except for flat losses, fixed frequency-response shaping needs to be added to the compression. With such a frequency-dependent compression system, the loudness of each element of speech in the impaired left ear represented in Figure 9–7 would, other things being equal, be restored to the same loudness (within the accuracy of the compensation) that it has in the normal right ear, which is the loudness it has in the normal dynamic range of hearing.

COMPRESSION AND THE OUTER HAIR CELLS

In Chapter 6 recruitment was described as a negative effect, a deficiency in the normal compressing action of the outer hair cells that allows the entire dynamic range of speech and music to be accepted by the inner hair cells. Electronic compression may be thought of as an electronic substitute for a normal physiological function that has failed (Hood, Berlin, Hurley, & Wen, 1996). Steinberg and Gardner's (1937) prescient comparison of recruitment with expansion, and their suggestion that compression be used to compensate for recruitment, was made purely on the basis of their observations of subject responses, but the physiological basis of these responses has now been established.

HEARING-AID FITTING

It should be clear at this point that the third element of signal processing listed at the beginning of this chapter—adjustment of the compression and of the frequency-response shaping to make the processed speech fit into the residual dynamic range of hearing of the individual subject—is as important to bringing speech elements into the audible dynamic range of hearing as the processing itself. A signal-processing circuit is not a black box that works equally well for any hearing-impaired subject.

If the speech band is to be shaped to fit the subject's residual dynamic range of hearing for speech over the frequency spectrum, that residual area of hearing must be known. It is defined in Figure 9–1 as the area between the threshold curve in SPLs and an equal-loudness contour anchored to the subject's preferred level for listening to speech. Measuring such a contour is difficult and time-consuming, but at least two computer fitting systems, FIG6 (1997), and ELCVIL, estimate individual equal-loudness contours from threshold audiograms. They are able to do this because a survey of previous studies of impaired hearing showed a systematic relationship between subject thresholds and equal-loudness contours at higher sound levels.

Both the FIG6 and ELCVIL fitting systems provide target values of hearing-aid gain at different input levels and frequencies, gain values that are chosen to shape the speech band to fit proportionately into the individual patient's estimated dynamic range of hearing over the useful frequency range. FIG6 provides curves of target gain vs. frequency at three different input levels; ELCVIL works in a similar way but was designed for a particular Resound hearing aid. An earlier version of ELCVIL required entering the patient's preferred level for amplified speech, but ELCVIL has been modified to include the FIG6 method of estimating overall gain. The two fitting systems provide very similar results.

Because estimates of the gain required for individual patients used by these fitting systems are derived from statistical averages, the calculated fitting almost always benefits from readjustment on the basis of the subjective responses of the individual patient. Such subjective adjustments should not be made casually but in an organized sequence using presentations of processed speech, and since the adjustments need to start from a reasonably accurate base, the initial calculation is vital.

OTHER APPROACHES TO COMPRESSION

There is a variation in compression processing sometimes referred to as AVC or *automatic volume control*. This kind of compression responds only to the longer term level changes of speech, such as would occur at different talker distances. It has slower attack and release times, measured in seconds rather than milliseconds, and it does not change the intensity contrasts between closely spaced elements of speech. Moore, Glasberg, and Stone (1991) designed a compression system in which an AVC circuit precedes fast compression, and compressors have been designed with attack and release times that vary with the rate of change of the input signal (Teder, 1993).

THE LIMITS OF SIGNAL PROCESSING

Signal processing that includes both compression and frequency-response shaping, combined with careful fitting, can restore all or most of the speech cues to audibility for many hearing-impaired patients. Speech recognition for such patients is sometimes improved dramatically by this kind of processing, but it is rarely restored to normal. The more severe the impairment, the further from normal is the likely result. Making a maximum of speech cues audible to the hearing-impaired listener is the first task of signal processing for hearing aids, but apparently it is not enough. Most people expect and get 20-20 vision from their eyeglasses, but hearing aids cannot provide as effective a correction. Hearing-aid processing is intended to make maximum use of a damaged cochlea; it rarely regains the performance of an undamaged cochlea.

ELECTRONIC SIMULATION OF HEARING IMPAIRMENT

Electronic simulation of the symptoms of particular hearing pathologies can determine whether those pathologies affect speech enough to reduce intelligibility for a normal listener. If the simulation does reduce intelligibility for normals, that is strong evidence—assuming the validity of the simulation—that the pathology being simulated is at least partly responsible for the loss of speech intelligibility by hearing-impaired persons. Processing to compensate that pathology would then be directed at the right problem. If the simulation does not reduce intelligibility for normal listeners, that is evidence that the pathology allows an adequate set of speech cues to remain audible and that the intelligibility problem lies elsewhere: for example, in an inability to decode speech cues, or in other hearing pathologies, perhaps in combination with the pathology that was simulated. Processing to compensate only for the pathology that was simulated would be misdirected.

A second use for simulations is to test methods of compensatory processing. The results of such trials, however, yield useful hypotheses rather than conclusions, and they must be tested in the real world of the hearing impaired.

Simulations of recruitment/high-frequency loss (Duchnowski & Zurek, 1995; Villchur, 1974, 1977) have shown that these pathologies, especially in combination, do erode speech intelligibility significantly. Recruitment was simulated in each study by a multichannel bank of electronic expanders; accentuated high-frequency loss was simulated by low-pass filtering (high-frequency attenuation). Villchur validated his simulations with unilaterally impaired subjects. Each subject compared the simulation (adjusted to the particular impairment) in his or her good ear with the real thing (unprocessed speech amplified to the same volume) in the impaired ear. Duchnowski and Zurek validated their simulations by analyzing and comparing the speech-test performance of normal subjects listening to the simulation with the performance of impaired subjects listening to amplified, unprocessed speech.

Simulation of the loss of frequency selectivity (Villchur, 1977) has suggested that frequency selectivity must be reduced substantially to affect speech intelligibility significantly.

THE COMPRESSION CONTROVERSY

The intelligibility scores of all six subjects of the 1973 Villchur experiment were increased by the processing in Figure 9–6, in quiet and in the presence of speech interference. Scores were more than doubled for some of the subjects.[5] Among the experimenters who conducted later compression studies, the only consensus has been that there is a lack of consensus. Some studies contradicted the Villchur results, some confirmed them, and others reached conclusions somewhere in between contradiction and confirmation.

Some authorities have stated that compression with short attack and release times has an inherent and predictable negative effect on speech recognition, especially in multichannel designs in which separate compressors control each frequency channel and when interfering speech is present. Their basic argument is that the reduction of loudness contrasts by compression compromises the "spectral integrity" of speech, by which they mean that compression changes the normal intensity contrasts between speech elements in different parts of the frequency spectrum. They say these contrasts are important to speech understanding. Plomp (1988) compared the reduction of intensity contrasts by fast multichannel compression to the effect of noise on the "modulation transfer function"[6] of a communication system, and predicted that such compression would have an effect on speech intelligibility comparable to the effect of noise. Noise, like compression, can

---

[5]The 1973 Villchur study has been criticized for not separating the effects of compression and high-frequency emphasis.

[6]The modulation transfer function is an index of the accuracy with which the amplitude contrasts in the wave envelope of a signal are preserved. Compression flattens the wave envelope by reducing intensity contrasts; noise has a similar effect by filling in the troughs of the envelope. But noise masks the low-amplitude elements of the signal represented in the troughs, while compression preserves them.

create a reduction of intensity contrasts by filling in the troughs of the speech wave envelope.

It is of course true that compression reduces intensity contrasts in speech, and that multichannel compression reduces the intensity contrasts between simultaneous speech elements at different frequencies. That is what compression is designed to do, in imitation of the original action of the outer hair cells. Compression compromises the spectral integrity of speech in terms of intensity contrasts, but restores this integrity to or toward normal in terms of loudness contrasts. Among the loudness contrasts that are restored by compression is the contrast between amplified elements of speech that are audible to the subject, and elements that remain below the subject's threshold of hearing even after uncompressed amplification to the subject's preferred overall level. To preserve the integrity of the above contrast in terms of intensity would require keeping the latter speech elements below the subject's threshold.

A detailed presentation of the theoretical objections to compression described above was given by Plomp (1988). An answer to Plomp by Villchur (1989), an elaboration of the answers given here, appeared in the same journal.

Several decades ago there was a controversy about binaural hearing aids similar to the compression controversy. Studies were published purporting to show no benefit from a binaural fitting, and the U.S. Federal Trade Commission issued a ruling (1971) that hearing-aid companies could not claim benefits for the use of two aids unless they accompanied the claim with a warning that many persons with a hearing disability in both ears would not benefit from using two aids. The warning was not justified. It is only under rare circumstances, such as the listener's inability to integrate signals in left and right ears, that a person with a hearing impairment in both ears does not benefit from binaural hearing aids. Today the binaural controversy has disappeared in the light of laboratory and clinical evidence, and I anticipate that the same will happen, one way or the other, with the compression controversy.

OTHER SIGNAL PROCESSING

Signal processing other than (or in addition to) compression and frequency response shaping has been designed to cope with more severe or profound hearing impairment: cases, for example, in which the subject has no usable mid- or high-frequency hearing. One system shifts part of the high-frequency spectrum of speech to a lower frequency range that is audible to the subject. There are also systems designed to extract and emphasize, or reproduce separately, speech features such as formants or fricatives. Surveys of these systems have been made by Pickett (1980) and by Levitt (1993). It should be pointed out that profoundly deaf persons typically have a severely reduced residual dynamic range of hearing (see Figure 3–5 of Chapter 3), and a processing scheme without compression would ignore the crippling effect of severe recruitment on speech intelligibility. Such processing might address some elements of the profound impairment effectively but would not address the overall problem (Villchur, 1978a).

Research in the area of radical signal processing for the profoundly deaf has largely given way to research in cochlear implants (which do use multichannel compression), and implants have had increasing success.

PROBABLE FUTURE DIRECTIONS IN HEARING-AID DESIGN

Predictions are always dangerous, but it is possible to speculate about the general direction hearing-aid design is likely to take, by comparing the path of hearing-aid research with the research that produced modern eyeglasses. Eyeglass design progressed from the use of simple magnifying lenses to lenses designed to correct for the myopia or hyperopia of the individual patient, and then to lenses that simultaneously corrected for these distortions and for astigmatism. The techniques and equipment designed to provide optimum compensation for impaired vision became more and more sophisticated and accurate, until today the great majority of people who use eyeglasses are justified in expecting their corrected vision to be normal.

The analogy between eyeglasses and hearing aids cannot be carried too far: Eyeglasses compensate for lenses of the eye that are deformed but typically healthy, while hearing-aid processing usually compensates for a damaged cochlea whose hair cells have degenerated. But the general direction of progress in hearing aids has been the same as in eyeglasses: first the discovery of the nature of the sensory deficit and/or distortion, and then the design of means to compensate, at least partially, for that distortion.

I believe that hearing-aid research will continue in this direction, that new and more sophisticated ways of discovering the nature of sensory hearing distortions significant to speech understanding will be developed, along with more sensitive and accurate ways of measuring the hearing distortions of individual patients. This knowledge will in turn allow the design of electronic circuits that compensate more accurately for individual hearing deficiencies, and such circuitry may require a complexity that calls for digital technology.

I think a second, parallel direction of progress in hearing aids will relate to the acoustical environment. Signal processing is not likely to restore normal hearing, so that hearing aids need to provide the impaired listener with a better than normal signal-to-noise and signal-to-reverberation ratio. Directional microphones and close-talking designs that do this are discussed in Chapter 10.

References

Allen, J. B. (1996). Derecruitment by multiband compression in hearing aids. In W. Jesteadt et al. (Eds.), *Modelling sensorineural hearing loss* (pp. 99–112). Englewood Cliffs, NJ: Lawrence Erlbaum.

American National Standard ANSI S3.22-1996. (1996). *Specification of hearing aid characteristics* (p. 11). New York: Acoustical Society of America.

Dix, M. R., Hallpike, C. S., & Hood, J. D. (1948). Observations upon the loudness recruitment phenomenon, with especial reference to the differential diagnosis of disorders of the internal ear and VIII nerve. *Proceedings of the Royal Society of Medicine*, pp. 516–526.

Duchnowski, P., & Zurek, P. M. (1995). Villchur revisited: Another look at automatic gain control simulation of recruiting hearing loss. *Journal of the Acoustical Society of America, 98,* 3170–3181.

Federal Trade Commission. (1971). Order, Docket 8791.

FIG6. (1997). *Hearing aid fitting protocol* [computer disk and instructions; includes ELCVIL disk]. Elk Grove Village, IL: Etymotic Research.

Hood, L. J., Berlin, C. I., Hurley, A., & Wen, H. (1996). Hearing aids: Only for hearing-impaired patients with abnormal otoacoustic emissions. In C. I. Berlin (Ed.), *Hair Cells and Hearing Aids* (pp. 108–110). San Diego, CA: Singular Publishing Group.

Killion, M. C. (1993). The K-Amp hearing aid: An attempt to present high fidelity for persons with impaired hearing. *American Journal of Audiology, 2,* 52–74.

Levitt, H. (1993). Future directions in hearing aid research. *JSLPA Monograph* (Suppl. 1), 107–124.

Moore, B. C. J., Glasberg, B. R., & Stone, M. A. (1991). Optimization of a slow-acting automatic gain control system for use in hearing aids. *British Journal of Audiology, 25,* 171–182.

Pickett, J. M. (1980). Frequency lowering for hearing aids. In H. Levitt, J. M. Pickett, & R. Houde (Eds.), *Sensory aids for the hearing impaired* (pp. 191–194). New York: IEEE Press.

Plomp, R. (1988). The negative effect of amplitude compression in multichannel hearing aids in the light of the modulation transfer function. *Journal of the Acoustical Society of America, 83,* 2322–2327.

Pluvinage, V. (1994). Rationale and development of the Resound system. In R. E. Sandlin (Ed.), *Understanding digitally programmable hearing aids* (Chap. 6). Boston: Allyn and Bacon.

Skinner, M. W. (1980). Speech intelligibility in noise-induced hearing loss: Effects of high-frequency compensation. *Journal of the Acoustical Society of America 67,* 306–317.

Steinberg, J. C., & Gardner, M. B. (1937). The dependence of hearing impairment on sound intensity. *Journal of the Acoustical Society of America 9*, 11–23.

Teder, H. (1993). Compression in the time domain. *American Journal of Audiology 2*, 41–46.

Villchur, E. (1973). Signal processing to improve speech intelligibility in perceptive deafness. *Journal of the Acoustical Society of America, 53*, 1646–1657.

Villchur, E. (1974). Simulation of the effect of recruitment on loudness relationships in speech. *Journal of the Acoustical Society of America, 56*, 1601–1611. [Recording bound in with article]

Villchur, E. (1977). Electronic models to simulate the effect of sensory distortions on speech perception by the deaf. *Journal of the Acoustical Society of America, 62*, 665–674.

Villchur, E. (1978a). The effect of a severely reduced dynamic range of hearing on the perception of speech. In C. Ludvigsen & J. Barfod (Eds.) *Sensorineural hearing impairment and hearing aids* (pp. 131–140). [Proceedings of the 8th Danavox Symposium; Recording bound in with article] Copenhagen: Danavox Jubilee Foundation.

Villchur, E. (1978b). Signal processing. In M. Ross & T. G. Giolas (Eds.), *Auditory management of hearing-impaired children* (Chap. 7). Baltimore: University Park Press.

Villchur, E. (1989). Comments on "The negative effect of amplitude compression in multichannel hearing aids in the light of the modulation transfer function." *Journal of the Acoustical Society of America 86*, 425–427.

Waldhauer, F., & Villchur, E. (1988). Full dynamic range multiband compression in a hearing aid. *The Hearing Journal, 41*, 29–32.

CHAPTER 10

Noise and Interference

Noise may be defined as nonperiodic sound, but it is also defined as any unwanted sound. The second definition is usually more suitable in audiological applications, because the interfering sound that plagues speech communication for persons with a hearing impairment may be speech or music.

Noise creates a greater reduction in speech understanding for persons with a nonconductive hearing impairment than it does for normal listeners. One reason such impaired listeners have a reduced resistance to noise is that they start out with a deficit in the speech cues they can hear in quiet, even after unprocessed amplification has raised the overall speech level to their preferred loudness. When noise takes out additional cues, they are left with a very sparse set of cues.

Experimental data have provided evidence that the reduction of audible speech cues in quiet is at least partly responsible for the special vulnerability of hearing-impaired persons to noise. When listeners with normal hearing were presented with speech that had been processed to simulate the loss of cues caused by hearing impairment, the normal listeners showed a greater than normal loss of speech understanding to interference, a loss similar to that of impaired listeners (Duchnowski & Zurek, 1995; Villchur, 1977).

After the deficiency in audible speech cues has been taken into account, however, hearing-impaired persons still have a greater than normal susceptibility to noise, a conclusion that we may again infer from experimental data: Making all or most of the important speech cues audible to impaired listeners helps them understand speech in noise, but it fails to provide them with normal resistance to the effects of noise on speech recognition.

Most of the research to improve speech intelligibility in noise for the hearing-impaired has consisted of attempts to improve the signal-to-noise ratio by separating the speech and the noise electronically. None of this processing has been consistently successful, because noise that is different enough from speech to be isolated and suppressed by an electronic circuit (such as the steady-state random noise the processing has usually targeted) is not representative of the noise encountered in real life. Another reason for the lack of success of electronic noise suppression is that the circuits that are designed to reduce the noise have tended to reduce speech cues as well.

Consider several people talking at the same time in front of a microphone or pair of microphones, and then consider the design requirements of a computer-controlled electronic circuit capable of separating the different voices and selecting the desired message. Such a circuit would have to respond to identifying cues such as voice quality, speech mannerisms, and the meaningful sequences of syllables and words: It would have to know not to combine the syllables and words of one speaker with those of another. It would also have to know which voice carried the desired message. These are analytical tasks far beyond the capabilities of a hearing-aid computer, yet the most common interference with which hearing-impaired persons must contend is just such interfering speech.

The computer in the human brain does have this capability. Broadbent (1958) described what he called the ability of humans to listen selectively: We can pay attention to a particular message among simultaneous competing messages. We have information in our memory banks necessary to the task—including a knowledge of the language—and a powerful computing capacity. As Killion (1993) has pointed out, the most powerful computer in the world can recognize a human face in half an hour, but a baby can do it in half a second.

The attention mechanism that makes selective listening possible requires a recognizable target message; we listen selectively by picking out recognizable patterns, or Gestalts, from the total sound. How, then, do we overcome the masking effect of competing signals on the target speech? We do it by taking advantage of the redundancy of speech cues. Coker (1974) called speech an error-resistant code because the code contains many redundant cues to its meaning. For example, speech that is cut off sharply above 2 kHz is readily understandable, but so is speech cut off below 2 kHz. The redundant cues of speech provide a reserve against the loss of cues to masking, making it possible for normal listeners to understand speech in noisy environments. But hearing-impaired persons do not hear many of the speech cues, even after undistorted but unprocessed amplification. The part of the speech they do hear may be enough for understanding speech in quiet, but when the impoverished set of cues available to them suffers a further loss from masking, there are insufficient cues left for them to fall back on.

It follows that the first line of electronic defense against noise is not to try to equal or outdo the brain's computer, but to process the signal to increase the number of speech cues available to the brain in quiet, so that more cues will be left after masking has taken its toll. Before attacking the daunting task of designing circuitry to reduce noise selectively, it makes sense to design circuitry to increase the resistance of the listener to noise by making more speech cues audible. Electronic noise suppressors typically do the opposite, by sacrificing rather than restoring speech cues.

This theoretical conclusion is supported by the experimental results of Villchur (1973). A combination of compression and frequency-response shaping, designed to increase the number of speech cues audible to each of six hearing-impaired subjects, improved the intelligibility scores of all six subjects listening in noise (2-voice speech interference 10 dB below the target speech signal), although compression made the overall signal-to-noise ratio worse. Compression restored the relative noise level to the increased level the subjects would have heard without recruitment, but the processing also increased their resistance to noise. For four of the six subjects, intelligibility scores were improved more by the processing than by eliminating the noise. Other experimental data (Moore, Johnson, Clark, & Pluvinage, 1992) have confirmed that restoring speech cues improves speech recognition in moderate noise. This approach by itself has failed, however, at high noise levels.

ACOUSTICAL MEANS FOR IMPROVING THE SIGNAL-TO-NOISE RATIO

Two hearing-aid designs have been successful in improving speech understanding in any type of noise at any noise level. Both use acoustical rather than electronic means to improve the signal-to-noise ratio.

One design is to place the microphone close to the talker's mouth rather than at the listener's ear (taking a cue from the old speaking tube), a system that dramatically improves the ratio between the level of the signal and that of any noise or reverberation. This scheme is effective but usually inconvenient except in special locations such as classrooms or theaters. In one system the microphone, held by the talker, communicates with the hearing aid by wireless transmission. The inconvenience of the listener handing a microphone to the talker may be well worth it in some cases of profound deafness. Telephone communication benefits from close talking, and the use of earphones connected directly to a television set provides a similar benefit.

A second design uses directional microphones that are less sensitive to sound behind them than to sound in front of them. In one type of directional microphone (Carlson & Killion, 1974), a single microphone has two ports of entry which lie on the line of intended directionality, and each port communicates with one side of the microphone diaphragm. As illustrated in Figure 10–1, side 1 of the diaphragm is open to the front microphone port, and side 2 is open to the rear port. When the instantaneous sound pressures on each side of the diaphragm are equal in amplitude and opposite in direction, the microphone has no output.

Sound from the rear of the microphone first enters the rear port. It is delayed by an acoustical network before it reaches side 2 of the diaphragm. The sound from the rear also enters the front port, but before it reaches side 1 of the diaphragm it is delayed by the time of travel between the rear port and the front port. The ports are spaced so that this time of travel is equal to the delay designed into the acoustical network[1] preceding side 2 of the diaphragm. Under ideal

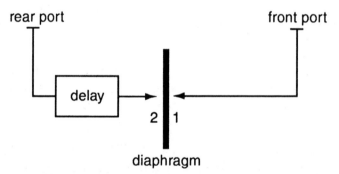

Figure 10–1. Block diagram of one type of directional microphone. An acoustical network between the rear port and side 2 of the diaphragm introduces a delay equal to the time it takes sound to travel from the rear port to the front port. For sound from the rear, sound pressures on the diaphragm from the rear and front ports are opposite in phase.

---

[1]The acoustical delay network introduces a phase shift approximately proportional to frequency, which makes the time delay of the network constant with frequency. The delay introduced by sound travel between ports is also constant with frequency. Therefore the delay network and port spacing can be designed for substantially equal delays over the frequency range of directional operation.

conditions the diaphragm is subjected to equal pressures from oppposite directions at the same points in the cycle, and the microphone has no response to this rear sound.

Sound from the front of the microphone first enters the front microphone port and is applied to side 1 of the diaphragm directly. Before it reaches side 2 of the diaphragm through the rear port, however, it is delayed twice: once in travelling from the front port to the rear port, and a second time in going through the acoustical delay network between the rear port and side 2. Because of these delays, at any given moment sound from the front reaches each side of the diaphragm at different points of the cycle. The instantaneous pressures on the two sides of the diaphragm are thus unequal, and sound from the front produces microphone output.

At low frequencies the delays that produce this microphone output are only a small fraction of the signal period, so that the differences between instantaneous pressures on each side of the diaphragm are small and microphone output is relatively low. As the frequency increases, the delays become a larger fraction of the signal period, and the front response of the microphone rises with frequency at 6 dB per octave. This rising response operates over the range in which the dimensions of the microphone are small compared to the wavelength of the sound being received. Since directional microphones are made small enough to be used with ITE hearing aids, the frequency limit on rising response does not amount to much.

In some directional microphones the rising response characteristic is compensated electrically. What cannot be compensated is the loss of microphone sensitivity accompanying the response characteristic, and other things being equal, directional-microphone systems have more circuit noise. However, the noisy environments in which directional microphones are needed are likely to cover up the internal circuit noise of the hearing aid. In some models of directional hearing aids the user can switch to standard nondirectional operation, which provides low circuit noise for quiet environments.

A directional microphone can show very high discrimination between front and rear sound when measurements are made in an anechoic chamber. But an anechoic chamber is not representative of real-life conditions; even the middle of an open field has reflections from the ground. In a normally reverberant environment, sound from the rear of the listener is reflected from room surfaces and will enter both microphone ports from all directions. Under realistic conditions a well-designed directional microphone of the type described above is likely to provide 4 to 5 dB of relative suppression of sound from the rear. This is a significant improvement in signal-to-noise ratio from the point of view of increasing speech intelligibility in noise.

Variations in directional-microphone design include the use of two separate microphones rather than the two sides of a single diaphragm for the cancellation function, and the use of an electronic rather than an acoustical delay network. When two microphones are used the cancellation takes place in their mixed electrical outputs, and an electronic delay circuit must work at the output rather than at the input of the rear microphone. The two microphone outputs must be matched; a drift in the relative sensitivity of either microphone will reduce the directivity of the system. In the single-microphone system a drift in microphone sensitivity does not affect directivity.

Persons with impaired hearing need all the help they can get for listening in noisy environments. Electronic processing that makes more speech cues audible, and acoustical methods of improving the signal-to-noise ratio, provide such help in different ways.

References

Broadbent, D. E. (1958). *Perception and communication*. New York: Pergamon.

Carlson, E. V., & Killion, M. C. (1974). Subminiature directional microphones. *Journal of the Audio Engineering Society, 22*, 92–96.

Coker, C. H. (1974). Speech as an error-resistant digital code. *Journal of the Acoustical Society of America, 55*, 476(A).

Duchnowski, P., & Zurek, P. M. (1995). Villchur revisited: Another look at automatic gain control simulation of recruiting hearing loss. *Journal of the Acoustical Society of America, 98*, 3170–3181.

Killion, M. C. (1993). The K-Amp hearing aid: An attempt to present high fidelity for persons with impaired hearing. *American Journal of Audiology, 2*, 52–74.

Moore, B. C. J., Johnson, J. S., Clark, T. M., & Pluvinage, V. (1992). Evaluation of a dual-channel full dynamic range compression system for people with sensorineural hearing loss. *Ear and Hearing, 13*, 349–370.

Villchur, E. (1973). Signal processing to improve speech intelligibility in perceptive deafness. *Journal of the Acoustical Society of America, 53*, 1646–1657.

Villchur, E. (1977). Electronic models to simulate the effect of sensory distortions on speech perception by the deaf. *Journal of the Acoustical Society of America, 62*, 665–674.

Author Index

Subject Index